Health Care Delivery Under Conflict:
How Prepared is West Africa?

Health Care Delivery Under Conflict:
How Prepared is West Africa?

Adedoyin Soyibo

UNIVERSITY PRESS PLC
IBADAN
2005

University Press PLC
IBADAN ABA ABUJA AJEGUNLE AKURE BENIN IKEJA ILORIN JOS KADUNA
KANO MAKURDI ONITSHA OWERRI WARRI ZARIA

ISBN 978 030 941 1
ISBN-13: 978-978-030-941-1

Published by University Press PLC
Three Crowns Building, Jericho, P.M.B. 5095, Ibadan, Nigeria
Fax: 02-2412056 E-mail: unipress@skannet.com
Website: www.universitypressplc.com

Contents

List of Tables   *x*
List of Figures   *xii*
List of Pictures   *xii*
List of Abbreviations   *xiii*
Acknowledgments   *xvii*
Dedication   *xix*
Executive Summary   *xx*

PART ONE: CONCEPTUAL ISSUES AND METHODOLOGY   **1**

CHAPTER ONE: **Introduction**   3
1.1   The Problem   3
1.2   Objectives of Study   4
1.3   Significance of Study   5
1.4   Study Methodology   6
1.5   Outline of Study   7

CHAPTER TWO: **A Review of the Literature of Post-Conflict**
                      Health Care   9
2.1   The Concept of Post-Conflict Health Care   9
2.2   Impact of Conflict on the Health System   11
         2.2.1   Impact on the Human Resource Base   13
         2.2.2   Impact on Policy and Management   13
         2.2.3   Impact on Physical Infrastructure   15
         2.2.4   Impact on Health Financing   15
2.3   Rehabilitation of the Post-Conflict Health System   16
2.4   Regional Dimensions of Conflict Management and Rehabilitation   17

PART TWO: SOCIO-ECONOMIC PROFILES OF STUDY
          COUNTRIES   **19**

CHAPTER THREE: Socio-Economic Profile of Guinea-Bissau   21
3.1   Introduction   21
3.2   Macroeconomic Performance   21
3.3   Health and Social Indicators   23
3.4   Burden of Diseases   24
3.5   Health Institutional Setup, Polices, Plans and Programmes   24

CHAPTER FOUR: **Socio-Economic Profile of Liberia**   28
4.1   Introduction   28
4.2   Macroeconomic Performance   29

4.3	Social and Health Indicators	30
4.4	Burden of Diseases	31

CHAPTER FIVE: **Socio-Economic Profile of Sierra Leone**   **33**

5.1	Introduction	33
5.2	Macroeconomic Performance	33
5.3	Health and Social Indicators	35
5.4	Burden of Diseases	36
5.5	Health Institutional Setup, Policies, Plans and Programmes	37

CHAPTER SIX: **Socio-Economic Profile of Cote d' Ivoire**   **40**

6.1	Introduction	40
6.2	Macroeconomic Performance	41
6.3	Health and Social Indicators	43
6.4	Burden of Diseases	44
6.5	Health Institutional Setup, Policies, Plans and Programmes	45

CHAPTER SEVEN: **Socio-Economic Profile of Nigeria**   **48**

7.1	Introduction	48
7.2	Macroeconomic Performance	49
7.3	Comparative Health and Social Indicators	50
7.4	Burden of Diseases	51
7.5	Health Institutional Setup, Policies, Plans and Programmes	53

PART THREE: POST-CONFLICT HEALTH CARE IN CONFLICT
              COUNTRIES   **59**

CHAPTER EIGHT: **Assessing Post-Conflict Health Care**
                         in Guinea- Bissau   **61**

8.1	Introduction	61
8.2	The Country: Guinea-Bissau and the Role of Government	61
8.3	Impact of Conflict on Health Care Facilities	68
	8.3.1 Characteristics of Respondent Facilities	68
	8.3.2 Effects of Conflict on Human and Other Resources and	
	Service Operations	69
8.4	The Roles of NGOs	74
8.5	Health System Performance	76
8.6	Summary, Implications and Recommendations	76

CHAPTER NINE: **Assessing Post-Conflict Health Care in Liberia**   **79**

9.1	Introduction	79

vi

9.2   The Role of Government   79
9.3   Impact of Conflict on Health Care Facilities   84
        9.3.1   Characteristics of Respondent Facilities   84
        9.3.2   Effects on Human and Other Resources and Service
                Operations   85
9.4   The Roles of NGOs   90
9.5   Health System Performance   93
9.6   Summary, Implications and Recommendations   94

CHAPTER TEN: Assessing Post-Conflict Health Care in
                     Sierra Leone   97
10.1   Introduction   97
10.2   The Role of Government   97
10.3   Impact of Conflict on Health Care Facilities   100
        10.3.1 Characteristics of Respondent Facilities   101
        10.3.2 Effects of Conflicts on Human and Other Resources
                Management and Service Operations   102
10.4   The Roles of NGOs   107
10.5   Health System Performance   110
10.6   Summary, Implications and Recommendations   110

PART FOUR: THE POTENTIALS FOR POST-CONFLICT
HEALTH CARE IN NON-CONFLICT COUNTRIES AND
REGIONAL HEALTH INSTITUTIONS   **113**

CHAPTER ELEVEN: The Potentials for Post-Conflict Health Care
                 in Cote d' Ivoire   **115**
11.1   Overview   115
11.2   Urgent Medical Aid Service (SAMU)   117
11.3   Groupment des Sapeurs Pompiers Militaires (GSPM)   119
11.4   Cross-cutting Issues   121
        11.4.1 Relationship between SAMU and GSPM   121
        11.4.2 The Relationship between Government Agencies
                and NGOs   121
11.5   Recent Experiences on Refugee Situations and Emergency
        Operations in Cote d'Ivoire   124
11.6   Conclusion   125

CHAPTER TWELVE: The Potentials for Post-Conflict Health
Care in Nigeria   127
12.1   Introduction   127
12.2   Overview   127
12.3   Existing Instruments and Agencies for Conflict/Emergency
        Management   129
12.4   Constraints and Limitations   140

CHAPTER THIRTEEN: The Role of ECOWAS and Other
Regional Health Institutions in
Post-Conflict Health Care   142
13.1   Structure of ECOWAS in Relation to Health Care Delivery
        Under Conflict   142
13.2   Conflict Resolution and Management Experience in West Africa
        and Possible Post-Conflict Health Care Effects   147
13.3   Assessing the State of Readiness of ECOWAS Health Institutions
        for Health Care Delivery Under Conflict   149
13.4   Future Roles for ECOWAS and Its Agencies for Health Care
        Delivery Under Conflict in West Africa   150
        13.4.1 Framework for Analysis   150
        13.4.2 The Proposition   151

PART FIVE: EPILOGUE   155

CHAPTER FOURTEEN: Looking Ahead–Implications of the Study,
Recommendations, and Conclusion   157
14.1   Summary of Findings   157
        14.1.1 The Socio-Economic Profiles of Study Countries 157
        14.1.2 Burden of Diseases   159
        14.1.3 Assessment of the Impact of Conflict on the Health
                System   160
14.1.4 The Role of NGOs Under Conflict   164
        14.1.5 The Role of Government Under Conflict   166
        14.1.6 The Potentials for Post Conflict Health Care in Cote
                d'Ivoire   169
        14.1.7 The Potentials for Post-Conflict Health Care in Nigeria 171
        14.1.8 The Role of ECOWAS in Post-Conflict Health Care 176
14.2   Implications of the Study and Recommendations   178
14.3   Limitations of the Study   180

14.4   Suggestions for Further Studies   180
14.5   Concluding Remarks   181

REFERENCES   **182**
INDEX   **187**

List of Tables

Table 3.1:	Selected Macroeconomic Indicators, Guinea-Bissau	22
Table 3.2:	Comparative Health and Social Indicators, Guinea-Bissau	23
Table 3.3:	Incidence of HIV/AIDS(1999), Guinea-Bissau	24
Table 3.4:	Health Facilities and Beds by Facility Category	25
Table 4.1:	Selected Macroeconomic Indicators, Liberia	29
Table 4.2:	Comparative Health and Social Indicators, Liberia	30
Table 4.3:	Incidence of HIV/AIDS in Liberia (1999)	32
Table 5.1:	Selected Macroeconomic Indicators, Sierra Leone	34
Table 5.2:	Comparative Health and Social Indicators, Sierra Leone	35
Table 5.3:	Department of Health Fiscal 1995 Expenditure	39
Table 6.1:	Selected Macroeconomic Indicators, Cote d'Ivoire	42
Table 6.2:	Comparative Health and Social Indicators, Cote d'Ivoire	43
Table 6.3:	Incidence of HIV/AIDS in Cote d'Ivoire (1999)	45
Table 7.1:	Selected Macroeconomic Indicators, Nigeria	49
Table 7.2:	Comparative Health and Social Indicators, Nigeria	51
Table 7.3:	Incidence of HIV/AIDS in Nigeria (1999)	52
Table 7.4:	HIV/AIDS Prevalence by Zone in Nigeria (%)	53
Table 8.1:	Effects of Conflict on Staff (Average No)	70
Table 8.2:	Effects of Conflict on Other Resources and the Management Process: Guinea-Bissau	71
Table 8.3	NGO Health Personnel During and After Conflict: Guinea-Bissau (Average No)	75
Table 9.1	Budget/Actual Expenditure of the MHSW, Liberia	82
Table 9.2	Projected Financing Gap in Health Sector Finance Requirements for Meeting the Targets Set in the NHP of Liberia	83
Table 9.3	Respondent Facilities by Type and Level of Care: Liberia	85
Table 9.4	Distribution of Conflict Duration in the Facilities in Surveyed in Liberia	85
Table 9.5	Effects of Conflict on Staff (Average No): Liberia	86
Table 9.6	Effects of Conflict on Other Resources and the Management Process (Average No/Amount): Liberia	88
Table 9.7	NGO Health Personnel During and After Conflict: Liberia (Average No)	92
Table 10.1	Respondent Facilities by Type and Level of Care: Sierra Leone	101
Table 10.2	Distribution of the Beginning and End of Conflict in the Facilities Surveyed	102

Table 10.3	Effects of Conflict on Staff (Average No)	103
Table 10.4	Effects of Conflict on Management Process and Other Resources (Average No)	105
Table 10.5	NGO Health Staff under Conflict in Sierra Leone (Average No)	109
Table 11.1	SAMU's Managerial Staff Structure (1996 – 2000)	118
Table 11.2	SAMU's Fiscal Position, 1996 – 2000 (CFA)	118
Table 11.3	GSPM's Managerial Staff Structure, 1996 – 2000	119
Table 11.4	GSPM's Fiscal Position, 1996-2000(CFA)	120
Table 12.1	Human Resources of Government Institutions Charged with Conflict/Emergency Care, 1960 - 1993	135
Table 12.2	Human Resources of the National Emergency Management Agency 1995 - 2001	136

List of Figures

Figure 8.1:   Conflict and Closure of Facilities: Guinea-Bissau   73
Figure 9.1:   Growth of Expenditure and Expenditure/Budget Ratio   82
Figure 10.1:   Conflict and Closure of Facilities   107
Figure 10.2:   NGO Type and Time of Establishment   108
Figure 12.1:   National Emergency Management Agency Organizational
               Chart   130

List of Pictures

Picture 8.1:   Part of the MINSAP Building Complex Used as One of
               the Head of State's Official Residences   64

Picture 8.2:   Part of the Hospital de Agosto in Bissau Destroyed During
               the War   65

Picture 8.3:   Annex of the General Hospital for Children Health Services 65

Picture 8.4:   LNSP, One of the Major Laboratories in the Country
               Which Was Badly Affected by the War   66

Picture 8.5:   A Part of the General Hospital Destroyed During the
               War   67

Picture 8.6:   Effect of the War on Another Part of the General Hospital 67

List of Abbreviations

A

ADB	–	African Development Bank
AFRC	–	Armed Forces Revolutionary Council
AHM,	–	Assembly of Health Ministers
AREF	–	African Refugee Foundation

C

CBOs	–	Community-Based Organizations
CBFA	–	Community-Based First Aid
CDC	–	Centre for Disease Control
CEPACS	–	Centre for Peace and Conflict Studies
CHTs	–	County Health Teams
COREN	–	Council of Registered Engineers of Nigeria
CSM	–	Cerebrospinal Meningitis

D

DALE	–	Disability Adjusted Life Expectancy
DFID	–	Department for International Development
DOH	–	Department of Health

E

ECOMOG	–	ECOWAS Ceasefire Monitoring Group
ECOWAS	–	Economic Community of West African States

F

FCT	–	Federal Capital Territory
FMF	–	Federal Ministry of Finance
FMOH	–	Federal Ministry of Health
FRSC	–	Federal Road Safety Corps
FY	–	Financial Year

G

GDI	–	Gross Domestic Investment
GDP	–	Gross Domestic Product
GDS	–	Gross Domestic Savings
GNS	–	Gross National Savings
GOL	–	Government of Liberia
GOROS	–	Government of the Republic of Sierra Leone
GPI	–	Gross Public Investment

GSM	–	Global System of Mobile Communication
GSMP	–	Groupment des Sapeurs Pompiers Militaires

H

HIV/AIDS	–	Human Immuno-Deficiency Virus/Acquired Immune DeficiencySyndrome
HRDP	–	Human Resources Development Plan
HSCC	–	Health Services Coordinating Committee
HSDP	–	Health System Development Project
HSF	–	Health System Fund
HSR	–	Health System Reform

I

IDA	–	International Development Administration
IDPs	–	Internally Displaced Persons
IFRC	–	International Federation of Red Cross and Red Crescent Societies
INCORE	–	Initiative on Conflict Resolution and Ethnicity

L

LASU	–	Lagos State University
LGAs	–	Local Government Areas

M

MCH	–	Maternal and Child Health
MCPMRPS	–	Mechanism for Conflict Prevention, Management, Resolution, Peacekeeping and Security
MHSW	–	Ministry of Health and Social Welfare
MIP	–	Maternal and Infant Protection
MINSAP	–	Ministry of Public Health

N

NACA	–	National Action Committee on AIDS
NCFR	–	National Commission for Refugees
NDRP	–	National Disaster Response Plan
NEMA	–	National Emergency Management Agency
NERA	–	National Emergency Relief Agency
NGOs	–	Non-governmental Organizations
NHA	–	National Health Accounts
NHAP	–	National Health Action Plan
NHP	–	National Health Policy

NHDP	–	National Health Development Plan
NHMIS	–	National Health Management Information System
NNGOs	–	Northern Non-governmental Organizations
NOCP	–	National Office of Civil Protection
NPFL	–	National Patriotic Front of Liberia
NPRC	–	National Provisional Ruling Council
NRCS	–	Nigerian Red Cross Society
NSE	–	Nigerian Society of Engineers

O

OAU	–	Organization of Africa Unity
OCCGE	–	Organization de Coordination et de Cooperation pour la Lutte Cent Les Grandes Endemies
ORSEC	–	Emergency Health Care Plan (Cote d'Ivoire)

P

PAHO	–	Pan- American Health Organization
PCASER	–	Programme for the Coordination and Assistance for Security and Development
PHC	–	Primary Health Care
PHUs	–	Peripheral Health Units
PLWA	–	People Living with AIDS

R

RCCI	–	Red Cross of Cote d'Ivoire
RDD	–	The Democratic Rally for the Republic
RDR	–	Rassemblement des Republicains
RUF	–	Revolutionary United Front

S

SAMU	–	Service d'Aide Medicale d'Urgence
SCH	–	Secondary Health Care
SHMB	–	State Hospitals Management Board
SMOH	–	State Ministry of Health
SSAs	–	Support Service Areas
STDs	–	Sexually Transmitted Diseases

T

| TAC | – | Technical Advisory Committee |
| TBAs | – | Traditional Birth Attendants |

U

UI	–	University of Ibadan
UN	–	United Nations
UNDP	–	United Nations Development Programme
UNHCR	–	United Nations High Commission for Refugees
UNICEF	–	United Nations Children's Fund
UNITA	–	Union for the Total Liberation of Angola
UNOMSIL	–	United Nations Observers Mission in Sierra Leone
USAID	–	United States Agency for International Development
USBs	–	Village Health Ports (Guinea-Bissau)

V

VHWs	–	Village Health Workers

W

WAHC	–	West Africa Health Community
WAHO	–	West Africa Health Organization
WASAM	–	West Africa Small Arms Moratorium
WHO	–	World Health Organization

Z

ZAR	–	Zone d'Accueil des Refugies

Acknowledgements

This study was supported by a generous grant from the Research and Writing Initiative of the Programme on Global Security and Sustainability of the John D. and Catherine T. MacArthur Foundation. I express my profound gratitude to the President, Management and the entire staff of the Foundation for giving me this rare opportunity. A number of other people contributed to seeing to the successful completion of the study. First, I will like to acknowledge the contribution of Professor Adigun A. B. Agbaje, Dean, Faculty of the Social Sciences, University of Ibadan, Ibadan, Nigeria; who first brought to my notice the existence of the Research and Writing Initiative of the Programme on Global Security and Sustainability of the John D. and Catherine T. MacArthur Foundation. Dr Adeboye Adeyemo, formerly of the Development Policy Centre, Ibadan, Nigeria; now of the African Capacity Building Foundation, Harare, Zimbabwe; was the Research Supervisor in Sierra Leone. Mr Victor A. B. Davies of the Department of Economics, Fourah Bay College, University of Sierra Leone, Freetown; was the Country Research Coordinator in Sierra Leone.

In Liberia, Professor Geegbae A. Geegbae, Chairman, Department of Economics, University of Liberia, Monrovia; was the Country Research Coordinator. Dr Kola Olayiwola, Head, Economic Policy Unit, Development Policy Centre, Ibadan; was the Research Supervisor in Guinea-Bissau. Mr Mario Cuhna, of the United Nations Development Programme, Bissau who was the Research Coordinator in Guinea-Bissau; was assisted by Mr Berhard Goubaly of the Taiwan Predio, Bissau. Prof. John C. Anyanwu, of the Department of Economics and Statistics, University of Benin, Benin City, Nigeria and the African Development Bank, Abidjan, Cote d'Ivoire; anchored data collection and also wrote a background paper on the potentials for health care delivery under conflict in Cote d'Ivoire. Dr Segun Ojo, Assistant Director, National Emergency Management Agency, Abuja, Nigeria; assisted in data collection and wrote a background paper on the potentials for health care delivery under conflict in Nigeria. Dr Tunde Alayande of the Economic Policy Unit, Development Policy Centre, Ibadan Nigeria; also assisted in data collection and wrote a background paper on the socio-economic profiles of the countries under study. I also acknowledge the contributions of the various countries' data collection teams. They were all wonderful!

Also acknowledged, are the contributions of participants at the workshop held to review the research design and instruments developed for the study in 2001 at the Board Room of the Development Policy Centre, Ibadan, Nigeria. Among them were Professor Adeniyi S. Gbadegesin, Dr Adeboye Adeyemo, Dr Tunde Alayande and Dr Kola Olayiwola. I have also benefitted from a number of international workshops and seminars organized by the Centre for Peace and Conflict Studies

(CEPACS), University of Ibadan, during my tenure as Dean, Faculty of the Social Sciences, University of Ibadan; particularly in relation to exposure to current data and literature on peace and conflict in Nigeria and in the West African subregion. In this connection, I thank the entire CEPACS team, led by the Director, Professor J. 'Bayo Adekanye, for this invaluable opportunity. I also had the opportunity of discussing health care delivery under conflict in Nigeria and West Africa with Ambassador Segun Olusola, Chairman, National Commission for Refugees, Nigeria and the Patron and Founder of African Refugee Foundation (AREF) as well as Chief (Mrs) Opral Benson, Chairman of AREF, during one of such seminars and workshops. Finally, I thank the Almighty God for giving me excellent health throughout the duration of the study and for His immense blessings always.

Dedication

To the millions of victims of the continuous civil strife in the West African subregion who suffer the indignity of poor Post-Conflict Health Care planning and delivery.

Executive Summary

This book is an outgrowth of the study of *The State of Post-Conflict Health Care Delivery in West Africa*, funded by the Research and Writing Initiative of the Programme on Global Security and Sustainability of the John D. and Catherine T. MacArthur Foundation. In the book, analysis of health delivery under conflict is undertaken within the rubric of post-conflict health care. This is because related health and development issues like relief, rehabilitation and reconstruction can be meaningfully discussed and better appreciated within post-conflict health care domain. And health, whether in peace time or under conflict, is a development issue.

Data for the study were collected by a network of researchers in the three conflict and two non-conflict countries selected for the study in 2001 and 2002. The three conflict countries are Guinea-Bissau, Liberia and Sierra Leone, while the two non-conflict countries are Cote d'Ivoire, representing Francophone countries and Nigeria, representing Anglophone countries. The broad objective of the study was to assess the state of readiness of West African countries in addressing issues of post-conflict health care, particularly issues relating to building sustainable national and regional human, material and institutional capacities for confronting, in a proactive manner, problems induced by conflict.

The specific objectives of the study are: the evaluation of the effects of conflicts on the health systems of the countries that recently experienced armed conflicts in the sub-region; examination and analysis of the ability of the existing human, material and institutional capacities of the health systems of West African countries to cope with the problems of post-conflict health care; analysis of the contributions of international agencies including non-governmental organizations (NGOs) to post-conflict health care delivery in West Africa; examination and analysis of the extent and effectiveness of the role of regional bodies like the Economic Community of West African States (ECOWAS) and its agencies like the West African Health Organization (WAHO) in post-conflict health care in West Africa; examination of the adequacy or otherwise of the legal and institutional frameworks for post-conflict health care at the national and regional levels in West Africa; and suggesting ways of building the necessary human, material, legal and institutional capacities for addressing the problems of post-conflict health care delivery in the West African sub-region.

The study used mostly survey data collected using four different instruments administered on Government/Administrative Agencies involved in Post-Conflict/ Emergency Health Care Delivery; Health Care Facilities; Non-Governmental Organizations (NGOs) involved in Post-Conflict Health Care Delivery; and Policy Makers. It also collected secondary data from government policy documents, guidelines and legal materials detailing the process and operation of health policy in each of the countries studied with a view to analyzing and assessing the state of readiness of the countries for post-conflict health care delivery. In this connection, the analysis paid attention to the existence or otherwise of the relevant institutional and legal frameworks for the management of conflicts and emergencies, and in relation to post-conflict health care delivery.

This book contains five parts. Part One which discusses *Conceptual Issues and Methodology*, contains two chapters. Chapter One, **Introduction,** motivates the study by defining the problem addressed, specifying the study objectives, and discussing the study methodology as well as discussing the significance of the study. On the other hand, Chapter Two, *A Review of the Literature of Post-Conflict Health Care,* reviews the concept of post-conflict health care, analyzes the impact of conflict on the health system, discusses the rehabilitation of the health system, and highlights issues relating to regional dimensions of post-conflict management and rehabilitation.

Part Two, *Socio-Economic Profiles of the Study Countries,* contains five chapters. This part found that the conflict countries are generally poor while conflict aggravated their poverty. In contrast, the non-conflict countries are relatively better off than the conflict countries in terms of GDP growth rate; though they have some areas of relatively poor economic performance. Health status in both conflict and non-conflict countries is, in general, low. Infectious diseases dominate the epidemiological pattern of the countries with malaria constituting a very high disease burden and this is aggravated by the existence of drug-resistant malaria. Other infectious diseases of public health concern include cholera, yellow fever and diarrhea.

Part Three, *Post-Conflict Health Care in Conflict Countries*, contains three chapters which assess health care delivery under conflict and in post-conflict situations in each of the conflict countries. The study found that the duration of conflict varied from one country to the other and affected health facilities differently. It lasted for about a year or so in Guinea-Bissau; seven to eight years in Liberia and nine or more years in Sierra Leone. In fact, conflict was still on-going in 7.7% of the facilities surveyed at the time of our field visit.

Conflict has negative effects on the human capital of the health system. In Guinea-Bissau, for example, before the conflict, there were, on average 2.30 doctors per facility. The number dropped by 50.4% to 1.14 per facility during the first year of conflict and marginally to 1.03 by 10% during the second year of conflict.

The supply of health personnel tended to improve with the cessation of hostilities. In Liberia, the average number of nurses per facility increased by over 120% from 9.11 to 20.1 between the first year after conflict and the second year after conflict. Conflict also leads to the destruction of health infrastructure. In Sierra Leone, the average number of functioning wards increased from 5.7 to 6.4 by 12% between the cessation of hostilities and the second year after conflict.

Conflict also has effects on service delivery at the facility level. In Guinea-Bissau, the average number of outpatients increased by 77.3% during the first year of conflict. During the second year of conflict, the average number of outpatients per facility increased by nearly 107.7%. Conflict has deleterious effects on the health management process too. In Liberia, with the onset of conflict, the average number of management meetings held per facility fell from 9.40 during the first of conflict by about 29% to 6.70 during the second year of conflict.

Another negative effect of conflict on the management process of health facility is the limitation on the maintenance function of the facilities' human capital. In the case of Sierra Leone, the average number of staff exposed to training per facility fell from 3.0 before conflict to 2.6 during the first year of conflict, a decrease of 13%.

NGOs are known to play important roles in health care delivery under conflict. A significant proportion of the NGOs appeared to be in operation mainly in response to the problems posed by conflict. In Sierra Leone, 41.2% of the NGOs surveyed started operation in the country after the commencement of hostilities. In Guinea-Bissau, the average number of health staff per NGO increased from 19 during the first year of conflict by 42.1% to 27 during the second year of conflict. NGOs also contribute to health care delivery under conflict through significant funding. In Liberia, for example, overseas development assistance to health care during conflict is characterized as 'robust in comparison to public sector spending'.

The role of government in health care delivery under conflict is affected by the level of institutional and policy framework in existence in the country as well as availability of financial, human and material resources to operate the system. In general, the study found that the Ministry of Health is the main government agency in charge of health care delivery both in peacetime and under conflict. All the study countries have at least one health plan or policy under which the health system operates. In general, all the conflict countries do not have specific guidelines or policy for health care delivery under conflict. Besides, there is no agency for coordinating the activities of development partners and NGOs during peace time or conflict. This can lead to wastages, duplications and inefficiency.

All governments of the conflict countries were adversely affected by shortage of funds and human resources to run the health system under conflict. In Guinea-Bissau, for example, the war aggravated its dearth of qualified personnel. Many of the health centres were without nurses, not to talk of doctors. The shortage of skilled manpower in the country's health system is also, in part, a reflection of the absence of tertiary and other professional institutions like a university for building such high human capital capacity in the country. Besides, in the West African subregion, except in the last five years or so, there is no institution for training and staff development in peace and conflict studies. In fact, so far, there is still none for training in health care delivery under conflict. There are two programmes at the Master's level in peace and conflict studies in the University of Ibadan, Nigeria and at the Diploma level, in Lagos State University (LASU), also in Nigeria. In relation to lack of financial resource during conflict, in Liberia, for example, the post-war health budgets of the Government of Liberia (GOL) were much lower than the pre-war budgets. Public allocation to health in 1981 was 10.2% of total budget. However, in 1990, during the war, it was 5.6% of a smaller national budget.

Part Four, which discusses *The Potentials for Post-Conflict Health Care in Non-Conflict Countries and Regional Health Institutions*, contains three chapters. In the first two of these chapters, the study shows that both Cote d'Ivoire and Nigeria have on ground some institutional and legal frameworks which can be scaled up to provide health care delivery under conflict. In Cote d'Ivoire two government agencies designated to provide emergency health care during conflicts or other forms of emergency are: (a) *the Service d'Aide Médicale d'Urgence*(SAMU), that is Emergency Medical Help Service and hence providing only medical services; and (b) The fire brigade, called *Groupement des Sapeurs Pompiers Militaires*(GSPM), a branch of the armed forces, which provides assistance during fire outbreaks, health emergencies and accidents. In the case of Nigeria, there are a number of government agencies as well as NGOs responsible for providing services under emergency, including health care services. These include NEMA, the National Commission for Refuges, the Armed Forces, NGOs like the NRCS and AREF. However, there are no explicit institutional and regulatory frameworks for addressing issues of health care delivery under conflict.

At the regional level, while there are no explicit institutional and legal frameworks for post-conflict health care, a number of protocols and treaties as well as regional health institutions exist which can be adopted and adapted to deliver health under conflict in the countries of the subregion. The establishment of a Mechanism for Conflict Prevention, Management, Resolution, Peacekeeping and Security(MCPMRPS), for example, as well as the signing of *Declaration of Moratorium on the Importation, Exportation and Manufacture of Light Weapons in West Africa*, commonly known as the West African Small Arms Moratorium(WASAM), provides a window of opportunity for such scaling-up. This is because MCPMRPS has been formalized in a way that led to the establishment of ECOMOG (ECOWAS Cease-fire Monitoring Group). It also allows for the broadening of ECOMOG to include military and civilian modules of Member States which can be creatively adapted to deliver health care under conflict.

In addition, ECOWAS has a regional health institution, the West African Health Organization (WAHO), which is expected to take-off through the merger of two other subregional health institutions. These are: the West African Health Community

(WAHC) serving Anglophone West Africa and *Organisation de coordination et de Cooperation pour la Lutte contre les Grandes Endemies*(OCCGE) which serves Francophone countries except the Republic of Guinea. As presently constituted, WAHO seems inadequate to address issues relating to health care delivery under conflict and/or in post-conflict situations. It is possible, however to adapt its features and characteristics like training, research and information dissemination, infrastructure as well as specialized human capacity, for building the necessary institutional framework for health care delivery under conflict and in post-conflict situation.

Part Five, *The Epilogue*, contains only one chapter which discusses the implications of the study, offers some recommendations and makes some concluding remarks. One major conclusion of the study is that conflict and non-conflict countries are not adequately prepared for health care delivery under conflict and in post-conflict situations. This, in part, accounts for exacerbation of the problems faced by the countries under conflict. Such negative experience may be repeated in non-conflict countries if they face similar problems. The study also established that at the regional level, ECOWAS and its agencies as presently constituted are also not well equipped to address the problems and challenges posed by health care delivery under conflict. However, the adoption of the MCPMRPS Protocol, offers a window of opportunity for adapting the existing framework to face these challenges.

It is my hope that this book will bring to the attention of the global audience the development issues emanating from poor health care delivery under conflict in West Africa, particularly as regards the insight it has provided into the conditions of the health systems of countries which recently experienced conflicts in the subregion. In this connection, all countries of the subregion and ECOWAS need to be proactive and plan well *ex ante* for meeting the challenges of health care delivery under conflict with a view to harvesting the benefits of good health care delivery under conflict, in the *unlikely* event there is one again! The experience of Cote d'Ivoire is instructive in this regard.

Adedoyin Soyibo
Ibadan
April, 2005

PART ONE

CONCEPTUAL ISSUES AND METHODOLOGY

Chapter One

INTRODUCTION

1.1 The Problem

There is a strong nexus between peace and development: peace promotes development and equitable development promotes peace. There are a number of local wars and intra-state armed conflicts in the world as of today. In Africa, the decade of the 1980s has been described as the lost decade. This has been due to the poor economic performance of the continent and its inability to keep pace with developments in various phases of human endeavours as has been the case in other developing subregions of the world like South-East Asia and Latin America.

The decade of the 1990s in Africa, which was characterized by a persistent and seemingly unending cycle of turmoil involving armed conflicts also became 'lost' to the dividends of development. Thus, there were armed conflicts in Somalia, Ethiopia and Eritrea which are in the horn of Africa; Sudan and Uganda in the East; Rwanda and Burundi in the Great Lakes region; the Democratic Republic of Congo and Congo Republic, in Central Africa; and Angola in Southern Africa. Besides, armed conflicts were experienced in West Africa during the decade in Liberia , Sierra Leone and Guinea-Bissau.

Wars and armed conflicts take their toll on human lives and destroy infrastructures like roads, bridges, educational institutions and health care facilities. Thus, they truncate the positive nexus between peace and development. Additionally, they lead to an influx of refugees on whom the additional trauma of lack of housing, adequate food, health care and the like, impose concomitant psychological and emotional strain. In fact, Luxen (1997) asserted that the psychological and emotional effect of war has been the most neglected impact of armed conflicts on human populations. The health system is one of those social systems, which are usually badly affected by crises and armed conflicts. Health systems often tend to collapse. In particular, most health problems that arise from conflict are as the result of the collapse of the human and material resources aspects of the health system in addition to the collapse of the economic, administrative and the political support provided by the state.

With the end of the cold war, local wars and intra-state armed conflicts have come to centre-stage in international affairs while the international community no longer takes the twin issues of peace and development in a fragmented fashion (Bush, 1998). A lot appears to have been done in this connection in relation to providing relief and rehabilitation of health and other physical infrastructures by foreign donors, multilateral agencies, and non-governmental organizations. In recent times, attention is shifting to the regional dimensions of peace-promotion, conflict resolution and management. This is important for a number of reasons. First, the impact of armed conflicts knows no national boundaries. Thus, an influx of refugees to neighbouring countries is often one of the first unintended effects of armed conflict in the subregion where the country experiencing conflict is located. Second, armed conflict can lead to regional instability as a result of the exacerbation of the socioeconomic, environmental, and developmental problems of the affected subregion consequent on the crisis.

Until very recently, most of the approaches and methodologies used in West Africa in resolving the problems created by armed conflicts, in general, appears *ad hoc* in nature and are often times externally-promoted. Besides, there appears to be a dearth of proactive regional initiatives, particularly as regards post-conflict health care delivery. Accordingly, a number of questions readily come to mind. In the countries that experienced conflict recently in West Africa, to what extent are their health systems affected? In general, how adequately prepared are the countries of West Africa for meeting the challenges posed by post-conflict health care delivery? What is the current stock of their human, material and institutional capacity for meeting these challenges? Are there efforts at the regional level for addressing the problems posed by post-health care delivery? If they exist, how adequate are they? How can post-conflict health care delivery be strengthened nationally and regionally in West Africa with a view to ensuring an equitable and sustainable development of the peoples of the subregion? These are some of the issues addressed by this study. However, as health, whether in peace time or under conflict is a development issue, analysis of health care delivery under conflict in the study was undertaken from the viewpoint of post-conflict health care. This is because from this perspective, related health and development issues like relief, rehabilitation and reconstruction can be meaningfully discussed and better appreciated.

1.2 Objectives of the Study

The study aims broadly at looking at issues relating to building sustainable national and regional human, material and institutional capacities for confronting, in a proactive manner, the problems induced by conflicts which adversely affect the health systems of the nations and health status of the peoples of West Africa. The objectives of the project are to specifically:

- evaluate the effects of conflicts on the health systems of the countries that recently experienced armed conflicts in the subregion;

4

- examine and analyze the ability of the existing human, material and institutional capacities of the health systems of West African countries to cope with the problems of post-conflict health care;
- analyze the contributions of international agencies including non-governmental organizations (NGOs) to post-conflict health care delivery in West Africa;
- examine and analyze the extent and effectiveness of the role of regional bodies like the Economic Community of West African States (ECOWAS) and its agencies like the West African Health Organization (WAHO) in post-conflict health care in West Africa;
- examine the adequacy or otherwise of the legal and institutional frameworks for post-conflict health care at the national and regional levels in West Africa; and
- suggest ways of building the necessary human, material, legal and institutional capacities for addressing the problems of post-conflict health care delivery in the West African subregion.

1.3   The Significance of the Study

This study is significant in a number of ways. First, it addressed issues relating to post-conflict health care, which are seldom spotlighted in peace and security studies in the sub region. By not addressing the issue is, in our view, a costly oversight, given the importance of health in the development process. In particular, in the case of people who are just emerging from the trauma of war, the condition of their health system and, concomitantly, their health status, can make or mar valuable efforts directed at ensuring reconciliation and equitable development.

Second, the study documented and analyzed the effects of conflicts on the health systems of countries that recently experienced them, with a view to bringing the status of these systems, in a comparative manner, to the global arena where they can easily receive help and assistance. Third, it evaluated the state of readiness of the national and regional institutions in the subregion as regards addressing the problems of post-conflict health, so that a proactive strategy can be developed in future to meet the needs of the countries of the subregion.

Fourth, the study identified lessons of experience in relation to post-conflict health care delivery with a view to putting more sustainable systems in place in future. Finally, by suggesting ways of building sustainable post-conflict health care capacity, the study contributed in no small way, to ensuring that the nexus between peace and development can be strengthened further in the West African subregion. This is because; reconstruction that follows rehabilitation can be enhanced faster with a strengthened post-conflict health care system, thereby leading to development, which can engender sustainability in the final analysis.

1.4 Study Methodology

The study involved an analysis of the existing national and regional capacities for post-conflict health care of the three countries that experienced armed conflict in West Africa in the 1980s and/or the 1990s, and case studies of two other non-conflict countries as well as ECOWAS and regional health institutions. The sample for the study included Liberia, Sierra Leone and Guinea-Bissau, as conflict countries; Nigeria and Cote d'Ivoire[1] as non-conflict countries, representing Anglophone and Francophone, respectively.

A survey of the state of the human, material and institutional capacities of the health systems of the conflict countries was conducted to assess the impact of the crises on the health care delivery system. This was done at two levels: governmental/administrative, involving mainly the central government and its institutions/agencies; and at the facility level. The latter was done by using a random sample of health care facilities, as much as possible, throughout each of the conflict countries under study, covering the primary, secondary and tertiary levels of health care delivery as well as both the public and private sectors.

Government policy documents, guidelines and legal materials detailing the process and operation of health policy in each of these countries were collected as much as possible and analyzed to assess the state of readiness of the countries for post-conflict health care delivery. In particular, the analysis paid attention to the existence or otherwise of the relevant institutional and legal framework for the management of conflicts and emergencies, and in relation to post-conflict health care delivery. Data were collected on the relevant human and financial capacities and other assets that can be used for emergency and post-conflict health care, if and whenever, the need arises. The performance of these institutions and their effectiveness in the delivery of post-conflict health care were also analyzed. Gaps were identified where they existed and suggestions for solving the ensuing problems were made. A semi-structured interview of top policy-makers was conducted to obtain their views on the effects of the conflict on the health system and how well equipped it is to deliver post-conflict health care effectively, particularly the ability of the system in coordinating the roles of the aid agencies and ensuring that the three rehabilitation dilemmas identified by Macrae (1997) are contained.

The international agencies involved in relief, rehabilitation, and reconstruction were identified and surveyed to assess their role and contributions to post-conflict health, particularly in the rehabilitation of the health system and in ensuring that the programmes they participate in are sustainable. In this connection, the study analyzed the extent to which such programmes address the issues of structural and infrastructural constraints of the system, whether they invest in human resource development or address issues relating to policy planning and management of the system.

6

In the non-conflict countries, the analysis only dwelt on assessing the potentials of the health system for providing post-conflict health care. Accordingly, data required were mainly secondary in nature and consisted of policy documents and guidelines · as well as laws and practices for combating emergencies particularly as they relate to health. This was done mainly at the central government level. The analysis also involved an evaluation of the human, material, institutional and legal capacities to confront the challenges posed by post-conflict health care, including the potential ability of the system to effectively coordinate the activities of donor agencies in such a way that they lead to sustainable development. Moreover, in addition, we attempted to analyze, the ability of the existing legal and institutional frameworks to ensure that the Macrae (1997) critical rehabilitation dilemmas could be contained.

At the regional level, the study analyzed the ability and potentiality of ECOWAS and regional health institutions to cope with post-conflict health care delivery in the subregion. Following Soyibo (1999), this involved analyzing their setup to determine and assess the state of readiness for conflict-prevention, resolution, relief and rehabilitation, particularly as it relates to post-conflict health care delivery. Second, it suggested developing relevant frameworks and methodologies that would build on the existing infrastructure of ECOWAS and these regional health institutions, and develop sustainable post-conflict health care delivery systems in member states. The data for these analyses were mainly secondary, and were obtained from documents, protocols, treaties, policies and guidelines of the various institutions.

Four instruments were specifically designed and used for the study for data collection in conflict countries:

- Instrument 01: For the Survey Government/Administrative Agencies involved in Post-Conflict/Emergency Health Care Delivery;
- Instrument 02: For the Survey Health Care Facilities;
- Instrument 03: For the Survey of Non-Governmental Organizations (NGOs) involved in Post-Conflict Health Care Delivery; and
- Instrument 04: Semi-Structured Interviews of Policy Makers.

Though, the secondary data were mainly collected for non-conflict countries, instruments 01 and 04 were used as guides for data collection in these countries

1.5 Outline of the Study
The study is organized in five parts. Part one, which includes this chapter, and one other chapter, which reviews the literature of post-conflict health care. Part Two, which contains five chapters, is concerned with a review of the socio-economic profiles of the study countries: the three conflict countries of Guineà-Bissau, Liberia

and Sierra Leone and the 'non'-conflict countries of Cote d'Ivoire and Nigeria. Part Three assesses health care delivery under conflict and in post-conflict situations in Guinea-Bissau, Liberia and Sierra Leone, while Part Four focuses on the potentials for health care delivery under conflict and emergency situations in Cote d'Ivoire and Nigeria. Part Five, where the study concludes, deals with attempts to look ahead and crystal-gaze, as it were, about the future of health care under conflict in West Africa; identify the implications of the study, discuss its limitations, offer suggestions for future research and proffer recommendations aimed at improving health care delivery under conflict in the subregion; and then draw conclusions.

---

[1] As at the time of the design of the study, there was no conflict in Cote d'Ivoire. Of course, Nigeria is known to have violent conflicts internally as in the case of the Niger Delta, as well as religious, inter- and intra-ethnic conflicts of various causes but mainly land-related or belonging to the genre of the so-called 'settler-indigene syndrome' and election-related political conflicts, among others: resulting in a number of internally displaced persons. These conflicts are becoming significant in recent times.

Chapter Two

A REVIEW OF THE LITERATURE OF POST-CONFLICT HEALTH CARE

We will first clarify some conceptual issues in health care delivery under conflict and in post-conflict situations. Then, we will review the literature as regards the impact of conflict on the health system, the rehabilitation of the post-conflict health system and the regional dimensions of conflict management and rehabilitation. These reviews formed the basis of our research design and implementation.

2.1 The Concept of Post-Conflict Health Care

Post-conflict situations tend to vary with context, time and space. The situations constitute a continuum. In some cases, post-conflict situations may involve transition from violence, to relief, to rehabilitation and to development, without recourse to violence again, at least not at a level that can undo all the post-crises achievements. This is exemplified by South Africa and Ethiopia. In others, there may be transition between phases of peace and crisis/violence resulting in the elongation of the relief and/or the rehabilitation phase of the post-conflict interventions. Liberia and Sierra Leone are examples of this type of situation. However, the presence of conflict/ violence must be at a level that will make the relief-rehabilitation and/or development intervention(s) both feasible and implementable. Accordingly, a post-conflict situation does not imply the total absence of violent conflict. Macrae, Zwi and Forsythe (1995a) identified four characteristic features of post-conflict situations.

- The signing of a formal peace agreement;
- A process of political transition by elections;
- Increased level of security; and
- A perception among national international actors that there is an opportunity for peace and recovery.

Not all these factors may be present simultaneously. Where there is a military takeover of power, for example, there may not be a formal peace agreement as was the case in Ethiopia in 1991 and Uganda in 1986 (Macrae, Zwi and Forsythe, 1995b).

In general, the process of post-conflict transition is highly unstable. Neither the signing of peace accords nor a change in the system of governance guarantees the permanence of peace. The process of political transition may bring with it new threats to stability. In West Africa, neither the signing of the Abuja Peace Accord on Liberia, the conduct of democratic elections and the installation of the administration of President Charles Taylor in the country, nor the reinstatement of the democratically elected president of Sierra Leone after the defeat of the rebels by ECOMOG completely guaranteed peace. In fact, recourse to violence in Sierra Leone began with the new year, 1999. Similarly, in Liberia, the recourse to violence intensified so much that a number of rebel groups emerged under President Charles Taylor. They ultimately ensured that he abdicated about six months to the end of his tenure and forced him to go into exile in Nigeria in August 2003.

In Afghanistan, the withdrawal of the Soviet army paved the way for an intensification of the struggle between the different factions of the Mujahadeen resulting in the emergence of the Talebans. In Cambodia, the Paris agreement and the UN-sponsored elections did not bring an end to the insurgency led by the Khmer Rouge. Despite UN-supervised elections in 1992 in Angola, UNITA was responsible for plunging the country into civil war after its defeat in the elections (Macrae, Zwi and Forsythe, 1995b).

One of the social systems which is most often adversely affected by conflict is the health system. The linkage, which the health system has with the health status of the populace as well as development, often makes it imperative to consider making restoration and rehabilitation of the health system a priority of any (post) -conflict relief and/or rehabilitation programme. Relief and rehabilitation can be conceived of as a continuum. The literature considers relief, rehabilitation and development as three important milestones of the post-conflict intervention continuum. These milestones also have inter-temporal equivalents. Thus, relief tends to coincide with the provision of short-term succour, often within a year involving survival assistance, while rehabilitation, which often overlaps with relief operations, is more concerned with the restoration of the war-torn system and the rebuilding of its infrastructure to save livelihoods. It is often targeted for completion within two years (DAC, 1997).

Macrae, Zwi and Forsythe (1995b) observed that in transitional situations, the rehabilitation task cannot be defined simply in terms of restoring the pre-conflict health system, since that health system is unlikely to be appropriate to the political and financial climate in the post-conflict period. Rehabilitation policies also have to take account of the need for, and in some cases the emergence of, new institutions and mechanisms for the financing and provision of services. It is also important to identify those adjustments, which are likely to contribute to the longer-term goals of sustainability and equity, and which threaten the achievement of these objectives. Given that in the transitional period, many of these adjustments take place largely outside government structures; it is important to identify ways in which new institutions can be supported and incorporated into the national health strategy.

Indeed, the rehabilitation process can be conceived as being made up of three inter-related elements (Kumar, 1997). These are:

- restoration, which involves bringing infrastructure and basic social facilities to functioning conditions;
- structural reform of the system leading to creating and/or dismantling organizations, institutions and administrative structures; and
- institution-building with a view to improving the efficiency and effectiveness of existing institutions.

Development operations are longer-term in nature, often extending beyond two years. They presume the existence of conditions of security and a functioning administration pursuing national objectives and strategies often in partnership with external actors (DAC, 1997). It should be noted that relief, rehabilitation and development operations are not necessarily sequential but may be carried out simultaneously.

Macrae, Zwi and Forsythe (1995b) asserted that with growing instability, the number and intensity of humanitarian crises around the globe has been on the increase. The crises have come to be described as complex emergencies. In this connection, the authors distinguished between disasters and emergencies. An emergency is defined by the presence of a hazard, whether natural or man-made. Whether an emergency leads to a disaster is determined by the coping capacity of a population or the individual. Thus, a disaster refers to a situation in which the capacity to sustain livelihoods and life are threatened by natural and man-made occurrences. When these disasters result from political factors, and in particular, high level of violence, Macrae, Zwi and Forsyth (1995b) describe them as 'complex disasters'. Given the level of violence resulting from political factors in West Africa in the 80s and the 90s, the case of the subregion in this period qualifies to be so described.

An effective post-conflict health policy and planning system for West Africa must take cognizance of the need to exploit to full benefit, the foregoing characteristics and interlinkages between relief and rehabilitation operations, on one hand and development operations, on the other. This will ensure the building of a proactive and effective response, relief, and rehabilitation post-conflict system *ex ante*, and hence improve the West African development landscape, if and when there is conflict. This study attempted to evaluate the extent to which the identified characteristics and interlinkages existed in the study countries.

2.2 Impact of Conflict on the Health System

Conflicts and violent crises have two types of impact on the health system: direct and indirect (Zwi and Ugalde, 1989, Macrae, Zwi and Forsythe, 1995b, Luxen, 1997). Many of the effects often linger long after the cessation of hostilities and violence. Direct effects are difficult to identify with certainty because they occur in a

11

deteriorated environment and are broadly related to military action. They include death, injury and physical and psychological disability of individuals, including health workers, and the destruction and looting of the health infrastructure, equipment and supplies (Macrae, Zwi and Forsythe, 1995b). However, physical (and direct) effects of violence like deaths, injuries and disablement as well as destruction of health infrastructure and equipment are often easier to identify and quantify than non-physical direct effects like psychological effects and mental pathologies (Luxen, 1997).

Of much greater magnitude, however, are the indirect effects of political, economic and social changes that both underlie conflict and precipitate it. For example, the risks of rape by military personnel, the increased levels of prostitution, which occur as female heads of households seek cash income in the absence of other productive activities and the breakdown of health facilities and the reduced opportunities for treating sexually-transmitted diseases (STDs) may increase the vulnerability of conflict-affected communities to HIV infection (Zwi and Cabral, 1991; Smallman-Raynor and Cliff, 1991; Bond and Vincent, 1990; and Macrae, Zwi and Forsythe, 1995b). Indirect effects of conflict on the health system, are often more significant in terms of aggregate mortality and morbidity and they include the impact of the general deterioration of the living conditions on hygiene, malnutrition and access to water (Luxen, 1997; Macrae, 1997). In this connection, women, children and the least economically privileged groups tend to be the most vulnerable to the negative effects of conflicts on the health system. Therefore, post-conflict health care interventions need to take cognizance of this identified impact of conflict on the health system.

Macrae, Zwi and Forsythe noted that conflict tends to exacerbate pre-existing structural weaknesses in the health system. However, its capacity to respond to the health needs of the people is reduced critically by the erosion of the capacity of the state in relation to finance, human resources, and managerial and organizational difficulties resulting principally from conflict. There is therefore, a need for a post-conflict health policy to plan the expansion of the health capacity in its rehabilitation efforts. Macrae (1997) suggested that this could be done in two ways. First, is the need for the rehabilitation of damaged infrastructure and/or the incorporation of health units that were out of government control in rebel-held areas and now in safe hands. Second, the expansion of the health system to include previously unserved populations as part of the process of peace building.

The four main types of impact that can be identified as confronting post-conflict health policy and planning as well as health care delivery under conflict situations are as follows:

- Impact on the human resource base of the health system;
- Impact on policy and management;
- Impact on physical infrastructure; and
- Impact on health financing.

12

2.2.1 *Impact on the Human Resource Base*

The public and private sector health care human resource base is usually adversely affected by conflict. Hostilities may lead to the migration of highly trained and skilled workers particularly those who are from other ethnic groups and so feel unsafe to work in areas other than where their ethnic groups reside. Thus, a combination of ethnic divisions, fear of reprisal, injury, hostage taking, and death affect the availability of human resources in conflict affected communities (Luxen, 1997; Macrae, 1997).

Such a situation often exacerbates the existing structural weaknesses in the health system like low level of support or supervision, weak logistic support, poor-quality training (Luxen, 1997) and the urban bias of health care delivery. Besides, the disruption of the educational system and the high level of poverty in the immediate post-conflict period, mean that fewer people are leaving secondary schools and entering university and other tertiary institutions (Macrae, 1997). This limits the availability of candidates for health personnel capacity building even in the medium term.

Besides, in developing countries like those in the West African subregion, there are usually no institutions for training and developing human capital for conflict resolution and management, as well as in peace and conflict studies, in general, and health care delivery under conflict, in particular. It is, perhaps less than five years and certainly less than a decade, since formal training in peace and conflict studies began at the tertiary level in Nigeria at the University of Ibadan (UI) and Lagos State University (LASU). In UI, there is a Master of Arts programme in Peace and Conflict Studies offered by the Institute of African Studies, which has been in existence for about four years now (2003). Also, in the same university, a professional Master of Science programme in Humanitarian and Refugee Studies, offered at the Centre for Peace and Conflict Studies (CEPACS) and sponsored by the Association of African Universities, began operation during the 2001/2002 academic years. In LASU, a diploma programme in peace and conflict studies has been instituted in collaboration with a Nigeria-based, international NGO, the African Refugee Foundation (AREF).

However, even with the existence of these training opportunities, there is still a general lack of training for specialists in health care provision both in under conflict and in post-conflict situations. The existing programmes may need to include, as part of their curricula, courses for specialists in post-conflict health care and also make deliberate efforts to develop and organize short courses to build the capacities of officials of government agencies and NGOs who will be involved in health care delivery under conflict as well as post-conflict and emergency situations.

2.2.2 *Impact on Policy and Management*

Perhaps, the greatest negative impact of the movement of health personnel from conflict-affected areas and the breakdown on financing of the health system, is the

13

depletion of the health system capacity for policy-making, planning and management (Macrae, 1997). Basically, management staff tend not to want to return to areas affected by conflict even after the cessation of crisis, given their bad experiences and perhaps, psychological traumas. In addition, the halting of training programmes due to funds shortage tends to aggravate the problem.

The whole debate on public health is usually brought to a halt and there is a general reversal of technical progress. Crisis can also have a negative impact on the political and administrative functions of the state represented by the Ministry of Health. In this regard, the Ministry may no longer be able to perform its functions with respect to maintenance of norms, as well as coordination, control and reforms. The lack of resources, particularly, human resources, together with political uncertainty, which is prevalent in the post-conflict period, make it impossible for the state to be reconstituted immediately. Thus, the planning and management aspects of health, are generally devoid of any substance at every level in the health pyramid, in the aftermath of crisis. There are inadequacies in key areas such as data collection, the monitoring of infections, resource planning, evaluation and supervision of programmes. Such inadequacies can only be remedied by reforms in the post-conflict period (Luxen, 1997).

Because of the breakdown in the policy institutions, there is often a crisis-approach to health planning. There is a breakdown in the lines of communication among the various stakeholders, as well as the referral capacity of the health care delivery system. There is disruption of routine disease monitoring and surveillance, disease prevention and control programmes as well as case findings and community care. There are also limited policy debates nationally and with development partners and multilateral agencies. Isolation of health facilities also becomes common, as a result of insecurity. The inability to collect and analyze data leads to a breakdown of the health information management system. Conflict also leads to a breakdown of civil institutions, such as the communities, which should normally aid health care delivery and as a result of the limited capacity of the health institutions in management, collaboration and networking. Consequently, there is internationalization of welfare provision (due to the influence of donors and northern NGOs), as well as entrenchment of vertical provision of service under a relief/rehabilitation model, accompanied by rapid, uncontrolled and undue fragmentation of service delivery into public-private cleavages. In fact, efforts aimed at reforms and privatization are usually consummated haphazardly and under undue haste (Macrae, Zwi, Forsythe, 1995b), perhaps because of undue external influence. Besides, the urban and curative bias of health care delivery that existed in peacetime becomes unduly exacerbated mainly because of the diversion of resources for the provision of acute and war-related care.

2.2.3 *Impact on Physical Infrastructure*

Some of the causes of the poor state of physical infrastructures in areas under conflict are destruction and neglect, lack of maintenance or no maintenance at all, dwindling financial resources, and looting. In addition, heavy and light equipment also tend to get destroyed and/or looted during violent crises.

Accordingly, vital hospital equipment like ambulances, beds and beddings, which can be easily looted if they are not destroyed, are usually in very short supply. Besides health system physical facilities, public utilities and infrastructures like water, telephone, roads and bridges are also destroyed in wars. The lack of these tends to inhibit an effective delivery of health care in the post-conflict period (Macrae, Zwi, Forsythe, 1995b).

2.2.4 *Impact on Health Financing*

Civil conflicts destroy physical and human capital, reduce savings and divert portfolio from domestic investments in order to avoid risk. This may lead to capital flight, and consequent negative financing and investment effects on the economy as a whole and the health sector, in particular. This often leads to frantic reduction in the health budget as result of distortion in the government expenditure, which then places more emphasis on defence spending in order to control unrest, rather than providing facilities that will improve human welfare. This will, in the final analysis, lead to reduced growth and increased poverty, which can lead to another cycle of violence (Ajayi, 2002). Other factors exacerbating the problem, are the privatization of finance and the provision of health care as well as the changing modalities of international support for health care financing (Macrae, 1997). In post-conflict situations in particular, the already weakened public health budget, is usually symbolically reduced to the payment of staff salaries alone, in most cases. In addition, there is usually a dearth of not only drugs and vaccines, but also of supplies. Luxen (1997) observed in this connection, that the whole social function of the state in its support for the population's health is called to question and then suggested that this explains why there is a need for reforms in relation to the new role the state has to play in the country's social future.

The consequences of this imploding of the welfare state are positive and negative. On the positive side, the reorganization of health service provision, financing and delivery, can make more health care accessible to the population through the emergence of profit and not-for-profit private sector (missions and NGOs), which increases service supply level, thus compensating for the vacuum left by the public sector. A second positive consequence is the creation of a greater sense of responsibility among communities and individuals in looking after their health. On the negative side, there may be an increasing restriction of access to the most destitute, the number of whom usually increases with conflict. Second, there tends to be a reduction in preventive and informative activities, and a tilt in emphasis towards curative care on account of its being adjudged more cost-effective, at least in the short/medium run.

Because of the conflict situation, governments tend to lay emphasis on war-related spending to the detriment of social sectors like education and health at all levels of the government, whether central, state/provincial, or local/municipal. As mentioned earlier, there is often a very high defence budget with a consequent reduction in the health budget, thus, there is greater dependence on external aid and increased importance of private financing of health financing, in spite of increasing household poverty brought about by the limited productive activities taking place in the economy as a result of conflict and limited access to cash by households.

2.3   Rehabilitation of the Post-Conflict Health System

The objectives of the rehabilitation of the post-conflict health system are to revitalize the most essential health activities, re-establish logistics and finance, and facilitate the re-establishment of the functions of the Ministry of Health (Luxen, 1997).

To achieve these objectives, Luxen proposed the following principles of activities:
- Identify problems and needs.
- Ensure that actions to be undertaken are suited to the specifications of the situation. Help create long-term sustainability, and take into consideration the most vulnerable population groups.
- Develop a strategy and a programme framework (Preferably managed by using the principle of the logic of proactive collaboration involving a team of specialists and in which NGO partners can find a place).
- Employ the principles of decentralization in implementing actions with institutional support and coordination being undertaken at the central and intermediate levels, while projects are undertaken at the level of first-referral hospitals and health centres (i.e. Specialists hospitals and health posts are excluded).
- As much as possible, ensure that relief-rehabilitation-development action plans are integrated and dovetailed into each other. This ensures that the rehabilitation phase gives priority to taking over from the relief phase in zones where security allows and where some level of structures exists. Reconstruction activities are then re-programmed as a function of new situations. Besides, institutional reforms are prepared during the rehabilitation phase and are executed as part of reconstruction activities.

Macrae (1997) identified three critical dilemmas, which confront the rehabilitation of health systems in post-conflict situations. These are: the dilemma of legitimacy of the transitional government; the dilemma of sustainability of rehabilitation; and the dilemma of coherence of rehabilitation policy and planning. The development of strong state institutions is very important to the achievement of the objectives of rehabilitating the health system in post-conflict situations. For example, if the human resource capacity development is to be increased, it will be important to work with civil servants, health professionals, and community representatives in order to improve their skill base and develop consensus on the direction of health policy for the future. This cannot be done effectively if the legitimacy of the government is in doubt. However, rehabilitation interventions are often implemented outside state structures and may not serve to strengthen them in the long term. This dilemma needs to be resolved.

In many cases, rehabilitation may not move beyond the relief-oriented and supply-driven approach. As conflict exacerbates the underlying weakness of the health system, sustainable rehabilitation must go beyond this short-term approach. It must involve a holistic analysis of the problems of the health system; identifying both its structural and infrastructural constraints; and invest in human resource development, and its policy, planning, and management systems.

Rehabilitation interventions in the health sector are often characterized by institutional fragmentation in financing and delivery of services. Typically, there is a host of actors- government, rebels, NGOs, and multilateral organizations, all doing different and sometimes the same things, in different places and often uncoordinated. This constitutes the dilemma of coherence. The mode of international assistance for health also changes during periods of conflict. In particular, Macrae, Zwi and Forsythe (1995b) noted that there is typically a shift away from supporting public provision and an increase in support for NGOs, particularly Northern NGOs (NNGOs) (Duffield, 1991; Hanlon, 1992; Macrae, Zwi and Forsythe, 1995b).

The proliferation of NNGOs in conflict–affected countries can result in important structural changes in the financing and provision of health services, often characterized by highly decentralized organization and management. The expanded roles of NGOs in this context, carries both risks and opportunities. Among the expected opportunities, is that community-based NGOs may be in a stronger position to promote the principles of Primary Health care (PHC), through training and community development activities. However, the relatively high costs associated with NGO-led relief intervention, and the difficulties of coordinating the different strategies they employ may not facilitate an easy transition to the development of a sustainable and coherent health system (Macrae, Zwi and Forsythe, 1995b). Therefore, ensuring coherent health planning is important, if the pattern of investment during the transitional period is to influence the longer-term prospects of health system development.

2.4   Regional Dimensions of Conflict Management and Rehabilitation[2]

Regional perspectives to resolving conflicts have heightened in recent years because intra-state violence has not only exacerbated socio-economic, environment and developmental problems, it has also raised the risks of regional instability. Accordingly, conflict management and rehabilitation, as well as prevention, require inputs at both sub-state and regional levels. Because of sovereignty and territorial integrity issues, post-colonial governments tend to resist outside involvement in situations of violent conflicts. However, they may be less averse to intervention(s) by regional bodies and agencies. This is perhaps the most compelling justification for working to strengthen regional approaches to conflict management.

The fact that internal conflicts generally produce instability at the regional levels means that effective strategies to proactively engage conflict situations will require coordinated regional approaches based on a commitment to agreed principles. The development of such a common set of principles is an essential first step. These principles should affirm commitment of member states to existing norms and standards defined by the UN and international law, and draw upon existing regional instruments. In particular, the end of the cold war has allowed the UN to reassert its Charter in promoting the use of regional arrangements as the preferred level of response to the preventive engagement and management of regional conflicts and post-conflict transitions.

Regional approaches (whether *ad hoc* multilateral contact groups or regional organizations) have an advantage in that they often accommodate sovereignty issues effectively by engaging state authorities in a process that is at once supra-state and localized. A government that is a member of a regional organization may feel less threatened by a regional process of engagement coordinated by that organization, than by non-regional factors. However, it must be noted that the impartiality of regional organizations and neighbouring countries is sometimes called to question. The case of ECOWAS Cease- fire Monitoring Group, ECOMOG in Liberia and Sierra Leone exemplifies this. Containment of domination and hegemonic fears, therefore, is important to ensure the success of regional intervention in conflict and post-conflict situations. Where there are regional struggles and hegemonic fears, wider international institutions may be more appropriate channels for international response and support.

While recognizing their potential, it is necessary to take cognizance of the limits of some regional organizations in the developing world. Many are financially-constrained and under-resourced institutions with little institutional or administrative capacity, comprehensive and integrated mechanisms for conflict prevention, peace-building and rehabilitation.

---

[2] This section borrows substantially from DAC (1997).

PART TWO

SOCIO-ECONOMIC PROFILES OF STUDY COUNTRIES

Chapter Three

SOCIO-ECONOMIC PROFILE OF GUINEA-BISSAU

3.1 Introduction

Guinea-Bissau is a small country located on the extreme south-west of West Africa. It covers a land area of 36,000 sq. km out of which 10.7 per cent is arable. It has a population density of 43 persons per sq. km. Its gross national income was $0.2 billion in the year 2000. It has an estimated population, which, in 2000 was 1.2 million people, with an average growth rate of 1.3 per cent between 1988 and 2000. Its major exports are groundnuts and palm-kernel. Guinea-Bissau suffered from years of civil war, which abated in recent times following the success achieved in holding the presidential and legislative elections in the country.

3.2 Macroeconomic Performance

The economy of Guinea-Bissau recorded one of the smallest growths in the subregion with real Gross Domestic Product (GDP) figures in the neighbourhood of only a couple of hundred million dollars (Table 3.1), averaging about $250 million over the review period. Gross Domestic Investment (GDI), Gross Public Investment (GPI) and Gross National Savings (GNS) as a percentage of GDP fluctuated over the review period and tended to decline, on average. For example, GDI and GPI, which were 22.3 per cent and 15.2 per cent of GDP in 1995, respectively, declined to 12.9 per cent and 6.2 per cent respectively in 1998 but increased respectively to 16.9 per cent and 10.8 per cent in 1999. Even in 1997, when government revenue as proportion of GDP was lower at 15.3 per cent, government expenditure and borrowing was as high as 46.3 per cent of GDP.

Guinea-Bissau also witnessed persistent depreciation of the local currency against the US Dollar over the entire period of review, although it was better than the situation in Sierra Leone. Besides, Table 3.1 reveals a mismatch in the sources and application of fund in the country. For example, total government revenue as a percentage of GDP was highest in 1999 at 17.3 per cent, while government expenditure and borrowing during this period was 31.3 per cent of GDP. The implication of this mismatch in the sources as an application of funds is the persistent deficit that the Guinea-Bissau economy recorded for the most part of the sampled period.

The external sector indicators of the Guinea-Bissau economy also paint a similar dismal picture as can been seen in the next table. Thus, the country persistently recorded deficits in its trade balance over the period under review. In terms of external reserves, the country can only cover four months of total imports, just 50 per cent of the African average of eight months.

Table 3.1: Selected Macroeconomic Indicators, Guinea-Bissau

Indicators	Unit	1995	1996	1997	1998	1999	2000
National Accounts							
GDP at Constant Prices	MnUS$	254	283	302	217	234	251
GNI per Capita	US$	220	230	230	160	170	180
GDP Annual Growth	%	4.4	11.6	6.5	-28.1	7.8	7.5
Gross Domestic Investment	% GDP	22.3	23.0	24.1	12.9	16.9	17.7
Gross Public Investment	% GDP	15.2	14.8	15.6	6.2	10.8	11.7
Gross National Savings	% GDP	4.7	6.6	9.4	-4.0	4.2	-2.6
Prices and Money							
Growth in Money Supply	%	47	51	236	-12	22	64
Exchange Rate	local currency/ US$	278.0	405.7	583.7	590.0	615.7	712.0
Government Finance							
Total Revenue	% GDP	12.7	12.5	15.3	5.4	17.3	19.6
Government Expenditure & Lending	% GDP	30.4	33.7	46.3	25.0	31.3	29.2
Government Deficit/Surplus	% GDP	5.2	-5.6	-12.7	-9.5	-3.3	-1.8
External Sector							
Current Account Balance	% GDP	-17.6	-16.5	-14.7	-16.9	-12.6	-21.1
Current Account Balance	MnUS$	-45	-45	-39	-35	-28	-46
External Reserves	Months of Imports	2	1	3	5	4	4
Term of Trade	Index	100	99.6	99.6	89.5	89.9	90.2
Debt and Financial Flows							
External debt Service	% of GDP	5.9	4.1	3.3	3.9	4.0	Na
Net Total Financial Flows	Mn US$	13	30	27	11	1	18
Net Transfers	Mn US$	7	26	23	7	-5	24

Source: *African Development Indicators, 1998 and 2002*
World Development Indicators, 2002
Note: *Na = Not Available*

3.3 Health and Social Indicators

The health system of Guinea-Bissau has, over time, suffered from various inadequacies, as regards personnel, funding, and supplies, among others. Its economic, demographic and other social indicators place it among the world's poorest. Life expectancy at birth was only 39 years in the 1980s compared to 42 and 48 in neighbouring Guinea and Senegal respectively (Table 3.2).

Table 3.2 : Comparative Health and Social Indicators, Guinea-Bissau

Indicator	Year	Guinea-Bissau	Africa
GNI per Capita (US$)	2000	180	671
Labour Force Participation Total (million)	2000	0.6	290.5
Life Expectancy at Birth (years)	1999	44	51
Infant Mortality Rate (per 1000)	1999	127	87
Maternal Mortality Rate (per 100,000 live births)	1999	910	734
Total Fertility Rate (Birth per woman)	2000	5.8	5.2
Population per Physician	1990-'99	5,665	Na
Population per Hospital Bed	1990-'98	677	1,133
Access to Safe Water (%)	1990-'98	53	56
Access to Health Services (%)	1995-2000	47	60
Percentage of Births Attended by Trained Health Personnel	1990-'99	50	43.7
Daily Calorie per Capita	1992	2,230	2,335
Public Expenditure on Health (% of GDP)	1990-'97	1.1	2.2

Source: *African Development Indicators, 2002*

The economic performance of Guinea-Bissau as reflected in the Gross Income per capita of US$180 shows that the country is relatively poor and the fact that it is much less than the African average of US$671 poses grave policy concern. The life expectancy of 44 years and the high infant and maternal mortality rates of 127 and 910 per 1000 respectively attest to the low health status in the country as a result of the deplorable state of the country's health system. These indices are much worse than the African averages of 87 and 734 per 1000 for infant and maternal mortality rates respectively. Though the population per hospital bed of 677 is a much better performance than the African average of 1,133; the population per physician is nevertheless very high and could account for the percentage of births attended by trained health personnel, which at 50 per cent is higher than the African average.

23

3.4   Burden of Diseases

The pattern of Guinea-Bissau's burden of diseases shows that communicable diseases, non-communicable diseases and injuries constitute the three main causes of morbidity and mortality in the country. Like most countries in Sub-Saharan Africa, communicable diseases of lower respiratory tract infections, diarrhea, tuberculosis and malaria account for about 38 per cent of the disease burden in Guinea-Bissau. Of considerable concern is that the incidence of tuberculosis, which is 361 per 100,000, is higher than the Sub-Saharan African average of 339 per 100,000 (World Development Indicators, 2002). The incidence of malaria is another source of morbidity in the country and accounts for between 20 per cent and 30 per cent of deaths with a large number amongst the by older children and adults range (Mcgranahan et al., 1999).

The burden of HIV/AIDS, another communicable disease, is slowly threatening the family fabric of the country. While 14,000 adults and children are infected by the disease, as many as 1,300 persons are estimated to have died of AIDS in 1999 (Table 3.3).

Table 3.3 : Incidence of HIV/AIDS (1999), Guinea-Bissau

People	Prevalence
Adults (15-49)	13,000
Adult Rate of Growth (%)	2.5
Women (15-49)	7,300
Children (0-14)	560

Source: *African Development Indicators, 2002*

Of greater concern is the fact that, women are the worst hit by the disease with an estimated infected number of 7,300 compared with 5,700 males. An estimated 560 children are also infected with HIV/AIDS. Besides, the cumulative number of children orphaned by AIDS in the country was estimated as 6,100 in 1999.

3.5   Health Institutional Setup, Policies, Plans and Programmes

The health system of Guinea-Bissau is organized around four levels of service provision at national hospitals, regional and district hospitals, health centres (clinics) and community-managed village health posts (USBs). There are two national hospitals, four regional hospitals, twelve sector (district) hospitals, 121 health centres and 450 village health posts (Table 3.4).

Table 3.4 : Health Facilities and Beds by Facility Category

Facility	Number of Units	Number of Beds
National Hospitals	2	633
Regional Hospitals	4	299
Sector Hospitals	12	279 .
Health Centres	121	-
Village Health Posts	450	-

Source: *Eklund and Stavem (1996)*

While the country has not developed any post-conflict health reforms policy like Sierra Leone, it continues to rely on the 1976 National Health Plan. However, the creation of 450 village health posts as shown in Table 3.4 is a reflection of the implementation of the country's National Health Plan. It emphasizes decentralization of services, preventive care (without neglecting curative services), and the use of simple techniques and practices. In terms of personnel, the plan underscores the educating and training of all personnel, including village health workers and village midwives who are volunteer staff.

The USBs were designed to receive assistance from the Ministry of Health in the form of construction materials, an initial stock of drugs, as well as supervision and training. They are entirely locally managed and staffed. Each USB is located in a standard two-room structure, which has been constructed with local materials (generally dried mud on a frame of branches or mud bricks), with one for 'general receiving' and the other, for patient care. The USBs administer simple treatment and basic drugs. Their inventory of drugs is restricted to twelve essential items and dressing materials. This tends to restrict the number of conditions and diseases they treat to cases such as malaria, diarrhea, conjunctivitis, cough, pain and wounds.

However, in terms of cost recovery, the Guinea-Bissau health system is based on the prepayment scheme in the villages (USBs) where healthy participants pay a premium in advance, for which they receive a free or reduced cost of health care if they fall ill. However, user-fee schemes obtain in health centres and hospitals where there seems to exist the greatest potential for resource mobilization from health care services in the country. The prepayment scheme, which allows for pooling of risks is beneficial to participants because it can help to prevent the catastrophe that may result from illness or injury. Ekmund and Stavem (1996) showed that prepayment schemes provide an equitable way to pay for care since the cost of treating illness is spread evenly over both the sick and the healthy. The rates and methods of prepayment vary substantially among villages in Guinea-Bissau. This suggests that, in the country, there is a high degree of autonomy at the village level in determining the payment

25

structure. For example, the annual fees paid per adult male varied from 20-500 pesos with a mean of 203.4 pesos. The average annual collection per capita in 1988, based on total population in each village, was 181 pesos, with a range of 28-981 pesos. Contributions to the prepayment scheme is done by adults who pay twice a year and are given receipts that serve as proof of membership, entitling them to free drugs and services at the time of each visit.

In terms of personnel, the USBs are staffed by one village health worker (VHW) and one midwife, both of whom are selected by the village political committee, whose membership is drawn from among the traditional birth attendants (TBAs), who provide prenatal care and perform deliveries. These midwives and VHWs have little or no education especially those who have been drawn from the rural areas and are trained for fifteen days by nurses at health centres and district hospitals. They are neither paid in cash or in kind for their time but they enjoy prestige and, in some villages, may be assisted with their agricultural activities, such as land clearing and/or harvesting. The Guinea-Bissau health system suffers from a dearth of qualified personnel with current ratios falling below the norm (Eklund and Staven, 1996). The authors also noted that except for medical doctors in national and district hospitals and auxiliary nurses, there are 1.3 physicians on average per health facility, against a norm of 2.7, and only 1.3 registered nurses on average, compared to the norm of 5.3. The situation in health centres is no different as there are just 0.5 registered nurses per facility, on average, compared to a norm of 1.1. The implication is that one out of two health centres is usually without a qualified nurse.

The Guinea-Bissau health system, especially the USBs, is based on community participation and a significant amount of local resources mobilization. In order to facilitate the smooth running of the USBs, there is always a letter of contract between the Ministry of Public Health (MINSAP) and the village leaders, which often defines responsibility as follows:

- the village decides on the fee levels for the prepayment scheme, whether payment is based per capita per adult or per household, and the timing of repayment;

- the village must collect funds under the prepayment system to ensure that initial drug supplies are continually replenished. Drugs are sold to USBs with substantial subsidies, set up at the central level and are equal across the region;

- some villages create special health sub-committees to oversee USB operations, but in the smaller villages, the responsibilities are performed by the political committees;

- the village provides the labour and most construction materials for building   the health post. MINSAP provides the windows, doors and hinges;

- the government supplies simple equipment, including a metal cupboard for storing drugs, stretcher, four chairs, one obstetrical stethoscope, one lantern, a kit of posters and other teaching aids, and an initial stock of drugs estimated to last for six months (for the population of each village); and

- the village selects one or more of its residents to be trained as VHW and midwives.

Chapter Four

SOCIO-ECONOMIC PROFILE OF LIBERIA

4.1 Introduction

Liberia is a small country, both in population and in geographical size. Before the outbreak of the civil war in 1989, the population of the country was only about 3 million, with a population density of 32 people per sq. kilometre as at the year 2000. It has a total land area of 96,000 sq. kilometre out of which 2.0 per cent is cultivable and about 36.1 per cent a forest area.

The Liberian civil war had its roots in the unique circumstances in which the country found itself. The country was established as a refuge for freed American slaves. It escaped the vicissitudes of European colonialism, only to be subjected to a harsh regime of 'democratic feudalism' imposed by a group of freed slaves, the Americo-Liberians, who perpetuated themselves as a ruling class for more than a century (Alao et al., 1999). The authors contended that the activities of this oligarchy, its termination, and the military regime that followed, all shaped the future of Liberia and served to explain the civil conflict that eventually engulfed the country.

Socio-politically, the people of Liberia are divided into two broad groups: descendants of the freed slaves, known as the Americo-Liberians, and the indigenous African population that had historically lived in the area. The former subjugated the indigenous Liberians after a series of wars from 1822 until the early part of the twentieth century. The ethnic composition of Liberia and the political tensions that developed as a result are central to understanding the country's civil war. The two main factors, which had long-term implications for the country, were: the self-perpetuating nature of the institutions and social structures that influenced the administration of Liberia, and the Americo-Liberian treatment of the indigenous population. Americo-Liberians constituted only 5 per cent of Liberia's population, and about 300 closely knit families formed the ruling elite. The activities of the Americo-Liberians have been well summed up by Wippman (1993):

> [They] created the social hierarchy they had experienced in the ante-bellum (of the United States) but with themselves as the socially dominant, land-owning class. They considered the indigenous population primitive and uncivilized, and treated it as little more than an abundant source of forced labor.

These remote as well as other imminent causes culminated in the vicious civil war that erupted in Liberia in 1989, especially with the attack of the Nimba county by a band of rebels known as the National Patriotic Front of Liberia (NPFL) led by Charles Taylor. Even after the Abuja Treaty and the installation of the civilian government led by Charles Taylor, the country has slipped back into civil war. All these underscore the need to assess the extent to which the health system of the country can withstand the stresses and strains of conflict.

4.2. Macroeconomic Performance

Even before the civil war, the Liberian economy had been under severe stress as it declined throughout the review period[1]. Also, Gross Domestic Savings (GDS) and Gross National Savings (GNS) as percentages of GDP, which fell in 1984, could not return to their 1980 values throughout the period of review (Table 4.1).

Table 4.1: Selected Macroeconomic Indicators, Liberia

Indicators	Unit	1980	1984	1985	1986	1987
National Accounts						
GDP at Constant Prices	MnUS$	1,265	1,180	1,170	1,151	1,189
GNP per Capita	US$	620	440	460	460	490
GDP Annual Growth	%	-4.5	-2.1	-0.8	-1.7	-1.0
Gross Domestic Investment	% GDP	27.3	10.2	8.7	9.7	Na
Gross Public Investment	% GDP	Na	Na	Na	Na	Na
Gross National Savings	% GDP	25.1	3.7	8.5	9.4	Na
Prices and Money						
Growth in Money Supply	%	Na	Na	Na	Na	Na
Exchange Rate	local currency/ US$	1.0	1.0	1.0	1.0	1.0
Government Finance						
Total Revenue	% GDP	18.1	20.4	18.9	16.7	15.9
Government Expenditure & Lending	% GDP	28.1	29.3	28.9	27.3	24.8
Government Deficit/Surplus	% GDP	-10.4	-11.4	-14.2	-12.1	-11.1
External Sector						
Current Account Balance	% GDP	4.1	-0.1	5.2	1.4	-10.4
Current Account Balance	MnUS$	46	-1	57	15	-118
External Reserves	Months of Imports index	0	0	0	0	0
Term of Trade	Na	Na	Na	Na	Na	Na

Debt and Financial Flows						
External Debt Service	% of GDP	3.8	5.4	3.3	2.7	1.4
Net Total Financial Flows	Mn US$	95	101	55	29	27
Net Transfers	Mn US$	60	69	30	11	16

Source: *African Development Indicators, 1998 and 2002*
World Development Indicators, 2002.
Note: Na = *Not Available*

Also, the total revenue as percentages of the GDP fell below the total expenditure throughout the period under review. The consequence of this is the persistent fiscal deficit, which the country witnessed.

The external sector performance of Liberia showed a precarious external reserve position, which was not enough to cover just one month of imports. The current account balance equally showed a dismal picture in 1987 as it declined to US$118 million as against the favourable balance of US$15 million in 1986.

4.3 Social and Health Indicators

Health and social indicators in Liberia indicate that the health status and the performance of the social sector have mixed results (Table 4.2). Thus, while life expectancy in Liberia is just the African average, the maternal mortality rate of 560 per 100,000 live births reveals a superior performance over the African average.

Table 4.2 : Comparative Health and Social Indicators, Liberia

Indicator	Year	Liberia	Africa
GNP per Capita (US$)	2000	Na	671
Labour Force Participation Total (million)	1998	Na	290.5
Life Expectancy at Birth (years)	1999	52	52
Infant Mortality Rate (per 1000)	1999	91	87
Maternal Mortality Rate (per 100,000 live births)	1999	560	734
Total Fertility Rate (Birth per woman)	1998	6.0	5.0
Crude Birth Rate (per 1000 live births)	1998	46.3	37.7
Crude Death Rate (per 1000 of the population)	1999	13.7	13.8
Population per Physician	1981	9,454	Na
Population per Hospital bed	1990-'98	Na	1,133
Access to Safe Water (%)	1994-'95	40	56
Access to Sanitation Facilities (%)	1995-2000	30	60
Percentage of births attended by trained health Personnel	1990-'99	Na	43.7

% of Under five suffering from wasting	1990-'99	Na	Na
% of Under five suffering from stunting	1990-'99	Na	Na
% of Under five suffering from underweight	1990-'99	Na	Na
Daily Calorie per capita	1992	2,067	2,335
Public Expenditure on Health (% of GDP)	1990-'97	Na	2.2

Source: *African Development Indicators, 2002*
World Development Indicators, 2002

However, the proportion of the population, which has access to safe water, and sanitation facilities of 40 per cent and 30 per cent, respectively falls below the African average of 56 per cent and 60 per cent, respectively. Infant mortality rate of 91 per 1000 is worse than the African average of 87 per 1000. Total fertility rate of 6.0 per woman is higher than the African average of 5.0 while the crude birth rate of 46.7 per 1000 live births exceeds the African average of 37.7 per 1000 live births. These figures tell on the limited resources available to government and households. It is no wonder then that the daily calorie intake of 2,067 in 1992 falls short of the African average of 2,335. Also the country's population per physician ratio of 9,454 in 1981 is much lower than the corresponding value of 15,241 for Cote d'Ivoire but higher than the values in Guinea Bissau (5.665 in the 90s) and Nigeria (5.208 in the 90s).

4.4 Burden of Diseases

The high prevalence of infectious diseases, which cuts across age profile and spectrum of the country, characterizes the burden-of-disease profile of Liberia, like most other countries located along the coastal parts of the subregion. Thus, Liberia is characterized by the prevalence of malaria, which is estimated to attack more than half of the population every year. It is one of the leading causes of death among under-fives and is of significant morbidity among the other segments of the society. The overall prevalence of onchocerciasis has not yet been determined. Other infectious diseases are cholera, yellow fever, and other epidemiological diseases like diarrhoea.

HIV/AIDS is another major source of communicable disease in the country. The national prevalence of HIV/AIDS by the year 2002 report was estimated at 39,000, which comprised adults and children. The spread of HIV/AIDS in Liberia is presented in Table 4.3.

Table 4.3 : Incidence of HIV/AIDS in Liberia (1999)

People	Prevalence
Adults (15-49)	37,000
Adult Rate of Growth (%)	2.8
Women (15-49)	21,000
Children (0-14)	2,000
AIDS Death	4,500

Source: *African Development Indicators, 2002*

Again, like most other countries in the sub-region, Table 4.3 shows that HIV/AIDS is rampant among women and represents about 57 per cent of adults with the disease. The estimated AIDS death of 4,500 is one of the lowest in the subregion. The table also shows that the AIDS pandemic also affects children representing about 5 per cent of people affected by the disease.

---

[1] The time series data for Liberia is constrained by dearth of data. The analysis is therefore based on the data that are readily available.

Chapter Five

SOCIO-ECONOMIC PROFILE OF SIERRA LEONE

5.1 Introduction

Sierra Leone is located on the southwestern coast of the West African sub-region and expands over a total land area of 71, 470 sq. km. out of which only 8.0 per cent is cultivated, 0.01 per cent constitutes forest and woodland while another 0.01 per cent is set aside for grazing. Its population, as estimated by the 1991 census, is 4.2 million with an average growth rate of 2.3 per cent per annum. While its mineral resources which include diamonds, gold, bauxite, rutile, among others, account for about 62 per cent of its GDP; its agricultural products include cocoa, coffee, palm-kernel, and ginger. Its export markets are USA, the European Union and other ECOWAS countries.

The political history of Sierra Leone is characterized by severe instabilities emanating from a long period of an inept and corrupt one-party civilian government that ruled the country for most of the post-independence period (Siegel, 1996). In April 1992, the military seized power and formed the National Provisional Ruling Council (NPRC) government, with a promise to stabilize and bring peace and prosperity within the shortest time possible. However, these hopes were never realized. In 1996, this led to a great insurgency, which disrupted the general social and economic activities in the country. The insurgency resulted in a change in the leadership of the NPRC, thereby leading to the holding of national elections, which were held in March 1996. The elections ushered in the new civilian government of Tejan Kabbah. However, the life of the newly elected civilian government would have been shortened by another coup *d'etat*, but for the intervention of the ECOWAS Cease-fire Monitoring Group (ECOMOG), which reinstated the government of Tejan Kabbah in Sierra Leone.

The conflicts engendered by these instabilities had devastating effects on the country in general and its health sector in particular. How did the health sector of Sierra Leone fare during these conflicts? What lessons can be learned from these experiences? As indicated earlier, such questions and more form the basis of this study.

5.2 Macroeconomic Performance

The economy of Sierra Leone fluctuated severely with an annual growth rate of less than 3 per cent between 1995 and 2000. In fact, growth actually declined in 1995,

1997 and 1999 by between 10 and 17 per cent (Table 5.1). Income per capita in the country is one of the lowest in the sub-region averaging $130 in 1999 and 2000. Gross National Savings (GNS) as a percentage of GDP declined for most of the period as Gross Domestic Investment (GDI) and Gross Public Investment (GPI) as percentages of GDP were less than 10 per cent throughout the period under review, primarily as a result of the civil war that engulfed the country.

Sierra Leone also witnessed persistent depreciation of its domestic currency against the US Dollar throughout the review period. Government revenue, as a percentage of GDP, also fluctuated widely. For example, government revenue, which was 8.6 per cent of GDP in 1995, fell to 5 per cent in 1997 and later increased to 12 per cent in 2000. The economy also suffered from large fiscal deficits with the government deficit as a percentage of GDP being as high as 10.4 per cent in 1998.

The external sector of Sierra Leone also recorded a dismal performance during the review period as the country persistently recorded a decline in its current account balance. The external reserve of the economy did not show any improvement throughout the review period as the country's external reserves could only cover less than five months of imports.

The war also impacted negatively on the exchange rate. It was 741.3 Leones to the US Dollar in 1995. By 1997, the Leone was exchanged at nearly 1,140 to the Dollar, declining to nearly 2,030 to the Dollar in 1998. The country also experienced high debt burden. Thus, the external debt service as a percentage of GDP was as high as 8 per cent in 1995, declining to 6.4 per cent and 5.9 per cent in 1996 and 2000, respectively. Besides, the net total financial flows also fluctuated. It was a net outflow of $136 million in 1995, rising to a net inflow of $44 million in 1996, but declining to $24 million in 1997 before rising again to $24 million in each of the years 1998 and 2000. However, there was a sharp decline to $20 million in 1999.

Table 5.1: Selected Macroeconomic Indicators, Sierra Leone

Indicators	Unit	1995	1996	1997	1998	1999	2000
National Accounts							
GDP at Constant Prices	MnUS$	962	978	812	835	740	792
GNI per Capita	US$	180	200	160	150	130	130
GDP Annual Growth	%	-10.6	1.7	-17.0	2.8	-11.3	7.0
Gross Domestic Investment	% GDP	8.5	7.4	5.2	4.8	5.0	3.4
Gross Public Investment	% GDP	7.4	2.3	3.1	3.0	3.0	1.8
Gross National Savings	% GDP	-0.5	-7.6	2.1	-3.1	4.3	-14.3
Prices and Money							
Growth in Money Supply	%	29	7	57	7	49	4
Exchange Rate	local currency/ US$	741.3	942.1	1,137.9	2,024.4	Na	Na

Government Finance							
Total Revenue	% GDP	8.6	10.5	5.0	7.4	6.8	12.0
Government Expenditure & Lending	% GDP	17.5	17.6	12.0	20.2	20.9	30.2
Government Deficit/Surplus	% GDP	-8.9	-5.3	-6.5	-10.4	-9.0	-9.8
External Sector							
Current Account Balance	% GDP	-7.3	-13.2	-1.2	-6.4	-3.7	-16.7
Current Account Balance	MnUS$	-70	-119	-11	-43	-26	-101
External Reserves	Months of Imports	2	1	3	4	3	2
Term of Trade	Index	100	71.4	71.4	71.4	77.3	72.3
Debt and Financial Flows							
External Debt Service	% of GDP	8.0	6.4	1.7	3.0	3.0	5.9
Net Total Financial Flows	Mn US$	-136	41	24	58	20	58
Net Transfers	Mn US$	-156	29	15	33	10	49

Source: *African Development Indicators, 1998 and 2002*
World Development Indicators, 2002

5.3 Health and Social Indicator

The nation's health system was under severe stress in the last decade due to chronic under-funding and neglect, thus the more than one decade of deteriorating health status indices of the people, characterized the health sector. Siegel et al (1996) noted that with declining government revenue, health expenditures were particularly hard hit as per capita health expenditures declined by over 85 per cent between 1980 and 1991. The World Bank (1996) also noted that in 1990, government spent 0.4 per cent of GDP on health care, less than 3 per cent of total spending, or less than US$1 per capital (Table 5.2).

Table 5.2: Comparative Health and Social Indicators, Sierra Leone

Indicator	Year	Sierra Leone	Africa
GNI per Capita (US$)	2000	130	671
Labour Force Participation Total (million)	2000	Na	290.5
Life Expectancy at Birth (years)	1999	37	51
Infant Mortality Rate (per 1000)	1999	168	87
Maternal Mortality Rate (per 100,000 live births)	1999	800	734
Total Fertility Rate (Birth per woman)	1999	5.9	4.9
Crude Birth Rate (per 1000 live births)	1999	45.1	37.2
Crude Death Rate (per 1000 of the population)	1999	25.1	14.5

Population per Physician	1990-99	Na	Na
Population per Hospital Bed	1990-98	Na	1,133
Access to Safe Water (%)	1994-95	34	56
Access to Sanitation Facilities (%)	1994-95	11	60
% of births attended by trained health Personnel	1990-99	Na	43.7
% of Under five suffering from wasting	1990-99	9	Na
% of Under five suffering from stunting	1990-99	35	Na
% of Under five suffering from underweight	1990-99	29	Na
Daily Calorie per Capita	1992	Na	2,335
Public Expenditure on Health (% of GDP)	1990-97	1.0	2.2

Source: *African Development Indicators, 2002*

Furthermore, Table 5.2 paints a dismal picture of the general socio-economic performance in Sierra Leone. The precarious health position of the country is further underscored by the different high mortality rates. The country had an infant mortality rate of between 168 per thousand live births in 1999; nearly double that of the African average of 87 per thousand live births. Life expectancy of 37 years at birth is equally worrisome given an African average of 52 in 1998.

The proportion of the population, which has access to basic services like health, sanitation and safe water poses a serious challenge to the health situation of Sierra Leone. While the percentage of the population with access to sanitation was 11 between 1990 and 1995, those with access to health services were 38 per cent in 1995. All these are lower than African averages, which are about 64 per cent and 58 per cent for health services and sanitation, respectively.

An examination of the public health expenditure as a proportion of GDP suggests limited commitment, at least, on the part of the public sector to revitalize the country's health sector, as regards funding. The table also shows that the public sector health expenditure, as a percentage of GDP was 1 per cent between 1990 and 1995, less than 50 per cent of the African average. The 1993 National Health Policy plan showed that this level of public sector health expenditure, made Sierra Leone the only country in the world with such a disproportionately low public sector health expenditure.

5.4 Burden of Diseases

Sierra Leone is characterized by a high prevalence of infectious diseases, which cut across the different age profiles and the social spectrum of the country. The only malariometric survey conducted in the country in 1977/1979 shows that the prevalence of 65.7 per cent of malaria makes it the leading cause of death among children under five and of morbidity among the other segments of the society (National Health

Policy Report, 1993). The overall prevalence of onchocerciasis has been recorded as 43 per cent (46% for males and 54% for females) in the forest – savanna mosaic of the northern region; and 85 per cent in the forest zone of the south.

HIV/AIDS constitute another major communicable disease burden in the country. The national prevalence of HIV/AIDS by the 1993 report was estimated at 4.7 per cent. Leprosy and tuberculosis have been estimated to occur at levels of 2 per 1000 and 103 per 1000, respectively. The epidemiology of schistosomiasis has not been satisfactorily determined according to the 1994 report, but estimates put its prevalence at 32.6 per cent of the total population (28.3% for males and 38.5% for females) for parts of a district. However, there are other diseases listed in the National Health Action Plan (1994) whose prevalence has not been measured at all in the economy like cholera, yellow fever and other epidemiological diseases like diarrhoea. All said and done the health situation in Sierra Leone, as depicted by the following disease burden patterns, should be a source of worry and concern for policy makers and researchers.

5.5 Health Institutional Setup, Policies, Plans and Programmes

In Sierra Leone, health care is provided by over 500 government health facilities, as well as 35 hospitals and 84 clinics that are operated by missions and the private sector. The government system includes 27 hospitals and about 400 peripheral health units including smaller community health posts in villages and larger community health centres in towns (World Bank, 1996). The Bank also noted further that much of the health system of the country was in disarray, with many facilities providing inadequate or virtually no services. Also of note was the observation of joint planning between facilities, and preventive and curative services.

However, the country has a post-conflict National Health Action Plan (NHAP), which is guided by an ideal vision of the health system. It was designed around twelve objectives, which were to be achieved through the integration of many vertical programmes, increased funding, decentralization of management, donor coordination, community participation, better training, and a redistribution of health facilities. However, the limitation of the availability of resources for the plan led to a refocusing of the twelve objectives around five major objectives:

- Improvement of maternal and child health;
- Prevention and control of communicable diseases;
- Nutrition;
- Improvement in sanitation and water; and
- Health information and education.

37

Following this action plan, a re-organization of health service provision, which focused on four main areas, was undertaken in the country. These four areas are (1) rationalizing the public sector facilities around delivery of a basic package of care; (2) developing human resources to manage and deliver health services in a more rational manner; (3) reforming the management of the Department of Health (DOH); and (4) developing partnerships.

In this direction, the DOH began to strengthen and redirect its delivery system with a strong emphasis on primary care delivered as part of a package of essential services. In this regard, Gibril (1995) noted that the Peripheral Health Units (PHUs) were to be the linchpin of these efforts with village health posts and larger health centres to be the main focus of the system. The basic package of clinical and public health services provided at the village health posts, health clinics and district hospitals were established along with a standardized equipment and drug lists needed to provide the services. The operational and financial management of these health posts, clinics and hospitals was devolved to the district level and hospital with each district having its own community boards.

In terms of human resources requirements, the personnel needs were to be met through a Human Resources Development Plan (HRDP). The manpower programmes highlighted new training of technical staff, and a new focus on management education and training, both at central and district levels. These were organized around two specialized training programmes to produce more staff for community health centres, village posts, and hospitals. The changes on the functions and training of staff was facilitated by parallel changes in the bureaucracy, which was partly designed to improve the incentives and working conditions of health staff in the public sector, while reducing the large numbers of non-service staff.

At the heart of the post-conflict health reforms in Sierra Leone was the change in the amount of allocation and the mechanism of financing and payment of health services provider. By 1994, the government of Sierra Leone had in this regard committed itself to raise social and health expenditures by 5 per cent per year, while the donor community committed itself to increase funding to meet the unmet needs of the core plans. The World Bank (1996) noted that the post conflict health reform witnessed a dramatic increase in government health expenditure as the government's national budget devoted to health was more than doubled in five years (2 per cent in 1990 to 5 per cent in 1994) (Siegel et al. 1996). Also, as a proportion of GDP, the authors noted that government health expenditure steadily increased from 0.4 per cent in 1990 to 1.0 per cent in 1994. A breakdown of the health expenditure in 1995 reflects the new priorities on prevention and primary care. Primary health care (PHC) received the lion's share of 31 per cent followed by support services with 25.7 per cent (Table 5.3). Support services include maintenance, administrative and planning cost at district levels. Drugs and medical supplies were allocated 17.2 per cent, followed by allocation to hospitals and laboratories (11.4 per cent). This is unlike previous situations where personnel expenditure usually predominates.

Table 5.3: Department of Health Fiscal 1995 Expenditure

Expenses	Funds (000's US$)	Per cent of Total
Primary & Preventive Service	7,024	31.0
Hospital & Laboratory	5,117	11.4
Drugs and Medical Supplies	3,897	17.2
Support Services	5,822	25.7
Others	797	3.6

Source: *Sierra Leone Department of Health, (1995)*

The involvement of key stakeholders in the post-conflict health reforms is another plus for the health sector revitalization in Sierra Leone. The stakeholders that have played an active role in the reform include:

- Community Representatives, who were based on formal settings, through the creation of standing health planning councils or committees at local levels and informal setting through ad hoc meetings and techniques as has been the case to date in Sierra Leone;
- The Department of Health is responsible for the implementation of the health reforms in the country;
- The Department of Finance is the administrative and budget unit from where the DOH draws its finances;
- Health Professionals include physicians and other non-traditional practitioners employed by the DOH. It also includes health service providers who saw health reforms as an opportunity to look at new delivery and finance systems;
- The Donor Community who provides the technical assistance, political support and financing needs of the health reforms; and
- The Academic Community who serves as invaluable catalysts or laboratories for health reforms and has helped increase accountability by publicizing data and benchmarks that might not be otherwise available.

Chapter Six

SOCIO-ECONOMIC PROFILE OF COTE D' IVOIRE

6.1 Introduction

Cote d'Ivoire is located on the south-central coast of West Africa and it expands over a total land area of 322,460 sq. km. out of which 9.3 per cent is cultivable and 13.8 per cent is permanently used for crop production. It had an estimated population of 16 million in the year 2000 and a population density of 50 people per sq. km, which is higher than the Sub-Saharan Africa average of 28 people per sq. km. Its Gross National Income per capita of US$600 in the year 2000 ranks it the 148th poorest country out of a total of 206 countries. Its natural resources include petroleum, diamonds, manganese, iron ore, cobalt, bauxite and copper while its agricultural products are coffee, cocoa beans (largest world producer), bananas, palm kernel, corn, rice manioc (tapioca), sweet potatoes, sugar, cotton, rubber, and timber.

Cote d'Ivoire has traditionally been a beacon of stability in the West African region, characterized by a relatively prosperous socio-economic situation and an infrastructure system that has benefited from extensive French development aid. However, since the death of former President Houphet Boigny, some degree of instability epitomized by political tension resulting from bottled-up ethnic rivalries surfaced in the country. In 1996, Bedie, his successor made some controversial decisions to contain perceived political rivals. He adopted the so-called "Ivorite" concept for determining eligibility of presidential candidates. Under this policy, only persons with both parents belonging to ethnic groups that were indigenous to the country could aspire to the country's highest office. Accordingly, he experienced a lot of opposition, which lead to a bloodless coup d'etat on December 24, 1999, led by General Robert Guei. Having lost state power, President Bedie fled from the country. The junta that took over did not help matters. Backed by some southern political leaders, General Guei added to the confusion. He continued with the controversial actions of Bedie and exacerbated tension. A second coup attempt in January 2000 failed and it was subsequently attributed to neighbouring countries of Burkina Faso, Mali and Guinea, thus generating more political and social tension. Finally, Alassane Dramane Ouattara, seen as the main target of the Ivorite policy –

and several other candidates – were banned from running the presidential ballot of October 22, 2000. Laurent Gbagbo, a southern politician, was the only contender of note perceived as being able to face the military and contain their excesses.

The stage was then set for a dangerous show down between northerners (mainly muslims and supporters of Ouattara) and southerners (mainly non-muslims). The presidential ballot took place as scheduled on 22 October, 2000 with a very low turnout of about 37 per cent. Ouattara's RDR (The Democratic Rally for the Republic) advocated a boycott. On 25 October 2000, Robet Guei attempted to hijack the election by cancelling the votes counted and proclaiming himself head of state. Laurent Gbagbo's supporters immediately challenged his move. They took to the streets backed by some army troops – (the Gendarmerie in particular) in Abidjan; San Pedro and Gangnoa in the Southwest; and Bouake in the centre of the country. A few hours of street riots were enough to topple Guei's military regime. However, on October 26, 2000, Ouatarra's supporters also took to the streets protesting the declaration of Gbagbo as President-elect and contesting even the electoral process itself. Chaos and confusion rocked the city of Abidjan. Churches and mosques were set ablaze by rioters while hundreds lost their lives.

To ease tension, Gbagbo initiated a Reconciliation Forum which was held from 8th October -20th December, 2001 and which was attended by the four major actors of the Ivorian political scenery: Bedié, Gbagbo, Guei and Ouattara. On 13th December, 2001 the forum recommended to the new political authorities to recognize Ouatara as a citizen of Cote d'Ivoire. During his closing speech to the Forum, Gbagbo declared that the question was to be handled by the Justice Department. On 22nd December, 2001, Ouattara introduced a request to the Justice Department for the deliverance of a national identity card, which has since been granted. Nonetheless, concerns remain about human rights situation and the democratic process while social justice still remains fragile. However, relations with the international community have resumed with France, the European Union, IMF and the World Bank granting financial assistance to the country.

Given the foregoing, and in spite of the fact that a full-scale war did not break out, these developments underscore the need to investigate how well prepared the country is for health care provision under conflict.

6.2   Macroeconomic Performance

Cote d'Ivoire, which has the largest economy of (CFA) zone of West Africa, suffered a severe setback in 1999 with growth rate of 1.6 per cent against 5.8 per cent in 1998 (Table 6.1). Its current account balance as a percentage of GDP fell to 5.42 per cent of GDP in 2000 from 3.9 per cent in 1999, largely as a result of a sharp fall in cocoa exports, higher oil import prices and reduced aid inflows. The depreciation of the Euro in 1999/2000, along with political turmoil in Cote d'Ivoire, led to the depreciation of the CFA against the US Dollar for most of the period under review. Government revenues also suffered largely because of low agricultural commodity prices and because the interim military regime also increased the government's wage bill in response to protests by soldiers and civil servants. The budget deficit/GDP ratio fell marginally from 2.9 per cent in 1999 to 2.2 per cent in 2000.

Cote d'Ivoire spends a significant part of its national income on debt service. Thus, as a percentage of GDP, debt service was 10.2 per cent in 1995 rising to 12.3 per cent in 1996, but declining marginally to 11.7 percent and 11.2 percent in 1997 and 1998, respectively and rising to 12.4 per cent in 1999.

Cote d'Ivoire has always enjoyed higher net total financial flows than most other West African countries, mainly because of the relative stability of the country. In 1995, for example, their net total financial flow was $0.94 billion, rising to $2.1 billion in 1996, but falling drastically to $0.41 dollars in 1997 and turning significantly negative, thereafter. In fact in 1998, at the height of the regime of President Bedie and rising discontent in the country, it fell to -$1.1 billion.

Table 6.1 : Selected Macroeconomic Indicators, Cote d'Ivoire

Indicators	Unit	1995	1996	1997	1998	1999	2000
National Accounts							
GDP at Constant Prices	MnUS$	9,992	10,681	11,322	11,978	12,170	11,800
GNI per Capita	US$	650	660	700	690	670	660
GDP Annual Growth	%	7.0	6.9	6.0	5.8	1.6	-2.3
Gross Domestic Investment	% GDP	16.4	15.6	15.8	16.4	16.0	14.1
Gross Public Investment	% GDP	5.6	5.5	6.0	6.7	4.8	3.6
Gross National Savings	% GDP	10.6	10.9	11.2	12.4	11.9	9.6
Prices and Money							
Growth in Money supply	%	18.1	3.9	8.2	6.0	-1.7	3.2
Exchange Rate	local currency/ US$	499.2	511.6	583.7	590.0	602.6	697.7
Government Finance							
Total Revenue	% GDP	22.8	22.9	22.0	21.2	19.2	18.4
Government Expenditure & Lending	% GDP	26.9	25.2	24.3	23.6	22.2	21.0
Government Deficit/Surplus	% GDP	-4.1	-2.2	-2.3	-2.4	-2.9	-2.2

External Sector							
Current Account Balance	% GDP	-6.7	-4.7	-4.6	-4.1	-3.9	-5.4
Current Account Balance	MnUS$	-668.0	-508.6	-490.1	-471.1	-465.1	-447.4
External Reserves	Months of imports	2.7	2.7	2.8	3.8	2.7	3.0
Term of Trade	index	Na	Na	Na	Na	Na	Na
Debt and Financial Flows							
External Debt Service	% of GDP	10.2	12.3	11.7	11.2	12.4	Na
Net Total Financial Flows	Mn US$	935	2,117	413	-1,064	-110	-191
Net Transfers	Mn US$	514	1,602	-109	-1,764	-66	-112

Source: *African Development Indicators, 1998 and 2002*
World Development Indicators, 2002
Note: Na = *Not Available*

6.3 Health and Social Indicators of Cote d'Ivoire

Cote d'Ivoire suffers the same declining health and social indices like the other West African countries considered in the study. The average life expectancy in the country is only 47.8 years, below the continental average of 52.5 years (Table 6.2).

Table 6.2: Comparative Health and Social Indicators, Cote d'Ivoire

Indicator	Year	Cote d'Ivoire	Africa
GNI per Capita (US$)	2000	600	671
Labour Force Participation Total (million)	2000	6.4	290.5
Life Expectancy at Birth (years)	1999	46	51
Infant Mortality Rate (per 1000)	1999	111	87
Maternal Mortality Rate (per 100,000 live births)	1999	810	734
Total Fertility Rate (Birth per woman)	2000	4.9	4.9
Crude Birth Rate (per 1000 live births)	1999	36.6	37.2
Crude Death Rate (per 1000 of the population)	1999	16.6	14.5
Population per Physician	1990-'99	15,241	Na
Population per Hospital Bed	1990-'98	1,250	1,133
Access to Safe Water (%)	1990-'98	65	56
Access to Sanitation Facilities (%)	1995-2000	Na	60
Percentage of births attended by trained health Personnel	1990-'99	47	43.7
% of Under five suffering from wasting	1990-'99	8	Na

% of Under five suffering from stunting	1990-'99	24	Na %
of Under five suffering from underweight	1990-'99	24	Na
Daily Calorie per Capita	1992	2,411	2,335
Public Expenditure on Health (% of GDP)	1990-'97	1.2	2.2

Source: African Development Indicators, 2002

The precarious health status situation in Cote d'Ivoire, well dramatized by its maternal mortality rate of 810 per 100,000, was one of the highest in the sub-region and was higher than the continental average of 234 per 1000 in 1999. Though population per bed of 1,250 is lower than the African average of 1,133, the population per physician of 15,241 is one of the highest in the sub-region and could account for the crude death rate of 16.6 per cent, which is higher than the African average.

The daily per capita calorie intake of 2,411 is high and is above the African average of 2,335. Access to safe water and the percentage of births attended to by trained personnel appear relatively satisfactory at 65 per cent and 47 per cent, respectively as they are higher than the African averages of 56 and 42.7 per cent, respectively. Although a comparison of child nutrition cannot be made because of paucity of data, 24 per cent of the under-fives suffer from both stunting and low birth weights whereas only 8 per cent suffer from wasting.

Also, like most other countries in the sub-region, the public sector health expenditure as a percentage of GDP of 1.2 per cent is quite low and is about 50 per cent of the African average of 2.2 per cent.

6.4 Burden of Diseases

An analysis of the burden of disease in Cote d'Ivoire reveals a high incidence of certain diseases that constantly put people off their daily activities. The average number of days a month in rural areas during which individuals could not pursue their normal activities was 7.5 for males and 7.9 for females compared with 5.3 days in urban centres (Gertler, 1990). Also, like most other countries in the sub-region, infectious diseases characterize the epidemiological pattern of Cote d'Ivoire, which has been worsened by malnutrition and high fertility in recent times. The epidemiological environment is dominated by the prevalence of malaria and other common diseases like dysentery, which has a prevalence rate about 400 per 1,000, pneumonia with a prevalence rate of about 130 per 1,000, and measles (WHO, 1999).

The World Bank (1994a) also noted that Cote d'Ivoire is characterized by such other endemic diseases like dracunculiasis, schistosomiasis and onchocerciasis, which are sources of illness and are associated with a loss of economic productivity. Tuberculosis, with a prevalence rate of 375 per 100,000 people and other water borne diseases like diarrhea and typhoid are also becoming diseases of serious public health concern due to the poor quality of health infrastructure and obsolete equipment. While the immediate cause of this situation is that the health infrastructure is not maintained; more profound causes however, lie in the paucity of public sector resources, the absence of a clearly defined health policy, and generally poor management in the entire field. The spread of the HIV/AIDS pandemic is another source of concern in Cote d'Ivoire. The total population with HIV/AIDS disease was 760,000 as at the end of 1999 (Table 6.3).

Table 6.3: Incidence of HIV/AIDS in Cote d'Ivoire (1999)

People	Prevalence
Adults (15-49)	760,000
Adult Rate of Growth (%)	10.8
Women (15-49)	400,000
Children (0-14)	32,000
AIDS Death	72,000

Source: *African Development Indicators, 2002*

The rate of HIV/AIDS growth of 10.8 per cent in Cote d'Ivoire is quite high and poses a very big policy challenge because it is higher than the African growth rate of 6.5 per cent. The estimated death of AIDS population of 72,000 is also quite alarming as it represents about 0.45 per cent of the total population of the country and almost a third of total AIDS deaths in Africa.

6.5 Health Institutional Setup, Policies, Plans and Programmes

The health care delivery infrastructure of Cote d'Ivoire is organized in the form of a pyramid. At the bottom are all primary health care facilities that include: public sector services such as urban and rural health centres; specialized primary health care centres; military health services; and the National Social Contingency Fund's medical and social services. Others are the miscellaneous preventive health care services connected to large public companies and institutions; private sector services such as private medical practices, laboratories, diagnostic imaging centres, infirmaries, and health services connected to private companies.

At the next level up, there are the referral services that include public sector services such as public hospitals and specialized clinics and private sector for-profit and non-profit services such as private hospitals and clinics. The Public Health Ministry includes specific agencies such as the Public Health Pharmacy, the National Blood Transfusion Centre, the National Public Health Laboratory, the National Public Hygiene Institute, and the National Health Workers' Training Institute.

The number of public sector health facilities rose from 700 in 1980 to 1,146 in 1996. In April 1996, the facilities owned by the Public Health Ministry included the following facilities: 218 rural health centres (all with dispensaries and maternity wards); 456 rural dispensaries; 5 rural maternity centres; one rural maternity and infant protection centre (MIP). Others are 23 area centres; 8 urban health units (all with dispensaries and maternity wards and MIP services); 124 urban health centres; 35 urban dispensaries; 14 urban maternity centres; 40 urban MIP centres, 49 school and university health services; 12 anti-tuberculosis centres; one mental health centre. The rest are 31 high school and college infirmaries; 7 prison infirmaries, 6 military infirmaries; 29 rural health bases; 56 general hospitals, 8 regional hospitals, 4 university hospital centres; 4 specialized institutes and two training institutes, etc. In the rural areas, there is one dispensary for every 10,000 inhabitants and one maternity centre for every 14,000 women of childbearing age.

Licensed private sector services include 25 private hospitals and clinics with 524 beds, 28 medical officers; 11 dental clinics; 82 companies with a health department; 383 pharmacies and 243 pharmacy warehouses; and 212 private infirmaries. With regard to the public sector medical and paramedical workers, the Ministry of Health Public Health survey held in December 1995 estimated a total of 16,536 of these classes of workers.

In terms of health strategies and plans, the fourth National Health Development Plan (NHDP) covering the period 196-2005 was adopted in April 1996. The plan's general objective, previously defined in the human resources development programme (PVRH), is to improve the health and well-being of the population by establishing a better balance in the amount and quality of service delivery to meet the population's basic needs. Its primary mission is to meet the demand for basic health services. To attain these goals, the NHDP established three more specific objectives:

- reducing the morbidity and mortality rates among the most vulnerable target population;
- improving the overall effectiveness of the health care system; and
- enhancing the quality of health services.

The first objective is to be achieved by promoting primary health care through the provision of a minimum package of services. The second objective is to render the health system more efficient and enhance the quality of health service by improving management. In particular, the programme to delegate responsibility and resources to regional and departmental directorates (health districts) will continue, research would be promoted, and the increased development and optimum use of human resources would be pursued with greater vigour. In addition, the government will also need to implement a bold national population policy to contain demographic growth and fertility, and to target sustainable human development.

46

In order to achieve its objectives, the NHDP has devised a number of strategies. In terms of high mortality and morbidity rates, it aims on the one hand to improve accessibility to services, and on the other, to promote the development of basic health care by implementing a minimum service package. To improve effectiveness, one strategy calls for better management of the entire health care system, encouraging a multi-sector approach, and better co-ordination between different service providers. Another strategy, with the end-goal of improving the quality of services recommends three tracks: (1) strengthening human resources in the health sector; (2) promoting research; and (3) developing health standards and improved health care system management.

In line with the Decree No. 84-721 of May 30, 1984, the Public Health and Population Ministry is, among others, responsible for:

- Creating, operating, and managing all health facilities in Cote d'Ivoire;
- Strengthening public hygiene and preventing widespread endemic diseases;
- Protecting mothers and children;
- Regulating pharmaceutical services;
- Organizing and managing private medicine and workplace health care;
- Training providers of medical or paramedical services (in conjunction with the Minister of National Education and Scientific Research);
- Contributing to the development and implementation of a national health policy;
- Investigating all medical problems related to immigrant and migratory communities;
- Addressing medical problems related to the family, especially the management of all public and private institutions, such as nurseries, day care centres, and kindergartens; and
- Preventing alcoholism, drug abuse, and mental illness.

A Public Health and Population Department, which is within the Ministry of Health, is responsible for:

- Monitoring the implementation of the nation's health policy, as well as the organization, technical control, and successful operation and management of the public health care system;
- Managing the practice of private medicine and health care in the workplace, including odontology and stomatology, in accordance with the law;
- Treating health problems related to demography, maternal and infant protection, and school medicine;
- Developing a primary health care strategy, organizing and managing the prevention of widespread endemic diseases; and
- Monitoring the activities of public health care facilities.

Chapter Seven

SOCIO-ECONOMIC PROFILE OF NIGERIA

7.1 Introduction

Nigeria is the largest country located on the West African region and expands over a total land area of about 924,000 sq. km of which only 31 per cent is arable and 2.8 per cent is permanently used for crop farming. It had a population estimate of 127 million in the year 2000 (World Bank, 2000). Its average population growth rate is 2.8 per cent per annum while the gross national income per capita of US$260 in 2000 ranks it the 186th poorest country out of 206 countries. While the country depends on crude petroleum as the main source of foreign exchange and revenue, agricultural exports include such crops like cocoa, rubber, and groundnut, among others. The country's main export markets are the United Kingdom, USA, other EU countries and other ECOWAS states, among others.

The phenomenal lack of trust among the federating units and different ethnic groupings in Nigeria is one of the major causes of conflicts in the country. In this connection, Benjamin (2002) argued that the Nigerian federalism is the derivation of rivalries between the major ethnic groups of Hausa, Igbo and Yoruba as well as between these dominant groups and the minority ethnic groups. Further, he argued that mutual suspicions and fears about one group dominating the other have been dramatically nurtured and heightened by self-seeking elites, such that instead of propelling a healthy competition for excellence, they tend to promote violent conflicts.

The current ethnic antagonism in Nigeria has reached crisis dimensions, assumed frightening heights, fuelling riots, accompanied by separatist agitations and sometimes violent extortions. Jega (1996) noted that the so-called 'elders' and 'opinion moulders/leaders', often opportunistically interested in the control of power and resources, usually pitch one region or ethnic group against the other with a view to positioning themselves for favourable bargaining positions in the body politic. The consequences of the foregoing are some of the various ethnic conflicts witnessed in different parts of the country recently. They include Zango - Kataf and the Hausa/Fulani crisis in Kaduna State; the Tiv/Jukun crisis in Benue State; the Ife/ Modakeke crisis in Osun State; the Ijaw/Itsekiri/Urhobo crisis in Delta State and the Aguleri/Umuleri/Umuoba-Anam crisis in Anambra State. Although these conflicts have not degenerated into full-scale wars, it is pertinent to seek to investigate the state of preparedness of the country in general and that of its health system in particular to address the problems such conflicts can generate, *ex ante*.

7.2 Macroeconomic Performance

The Nigerian economy has suffered from stagnation in recent times. The annual growth of GDP was only 1.1 per cent in 1999, much below the African average of 3.3 per cent (Table7.1).

Table 7.1: Selected Macroeconomic Indicators, Nigeria

Indicators	Unit	1995	1996	1997	1998	1999	2000
National Accounts							
GDP at Constant Prices	MnUS$	28,109	29,318	30,109	30,685	31,012	32,184
GNI per Capita	US$	210	250	270	260	250	260
GDP Annual Growth	%	2.5	4.3	2.7	1.9	1.1	3.8
Gross Domestic Investment	% GDP	16.3	14.2	17.4	24.1	23.4	22.7
Gross Public Investment	% GDP	5.3	5.2	7.1	11.3	10.4	9.8
Gross National Savings	% GDP	0.0	0.0	0.0	0.0	13.9	27.6
Prices and Money							
Growth in Money Supply	%	16	14	17	19	22	62
Exchange Rate	local currency/ US$	21.9	21.9	21.9	21.9	92.3	101.7
Government Finance							
Total Revenue	% GDP	22.6	19.7	20.0	16.2	30.7	46.1
Government Expenditure & Lending	% GDP	12.7	10.6	19.0	25.5	38.2	43.9
Government Deficit/Surplus	% GDP	13.6	11.4	3.5	-6.3	0.8	9.7
External Sector							
Current Account Balance	% GDP	-3.2	11.2	7.8	-9.6	-9.5	4.9
Current Account Balance	MnUS$	-897	3,953	2,840	-3,075	-3,290	2,003
External Reserves	Months of Imports	2	4	6	5	Na	5
Term of Trade	Index	Na	Na	Na	Na	Na	Na
Debt and Financial Flows							
External Debt Service	% of GDP	6.3	7.0	3.8	4.0	2.5	NA
Net Total Financial Flows	Mn US$	-559	-1,327	-663	-269	-2,031	-1,207
Net Transfers	Mn US$	-1,474	-2,418	-1,239	-826	-2,348	-2,038

Source: *African Development Indicators, 1998 and 2002*
World Development Indicators, 2002
Note: Na = *Not Available*

49

Gross National Income per capita of US$260 is lower than the African average of about US$650. Gross Domestic Investment (GDI) and Gross Public Investment (GPI) fluctuated throughout the review period, while Gross National savings was zero for most of the review period.

The official exchange rate to the US Dollar, which was fixed officially at 21.9 Naira, experienced a large depreciation in 1999 and in the year 2000 when it was liberalized. Also, total government expenditure as a percentage of GDP was lower than total revenue as a percentage of GDP, but in 1998, it shot above total revenue. For example, while total revenue, as a percentage of GDP was 16.2 per cent in 1998, total government expenditure as a percentage of GDP was as high as 25.5 per cent, resulting in a deficit of 6.3 per cent as a proportion of GDP.

The external sector did not fare any better especially when one considers the fact that Nigeria consistently witnessed a decline in trade balance for most of the period under review. For example, the current account balance as a percentage of GDP, which was 3.2 per cent in 1995, declined to 9.6 per cent in 1999. The external reserve covered imports from two months in 1995 to six months in 1997 and declined again in 1998.

In terms of debt servicing and net financial flows, Table 7.1 shows that external debt servicing as a percentage of GDP fluctuated during the review period. For example, external debt service payment as percentage of GDP that was 6.3 per cent in 1995 declined to 3.8 per cent by 1997, only to increase to 4.0 per cent by 1998. The net total financial flows paint a gory picture of a country that appears fleeced by a massive outflow of funds with net transfers of more than $2 billion in some as in 1996, 1999 and 2000, for example. The lack of capital inflows may not be unconnected with the pariah status of the country during most of the review period.

7.3 Comparative Health and Social Indicators

Nigeria witnessed a declining health status in the 1990s and more so in the last five years. The life expectancy of 46 years for the average Nigerian is below the African average of 51 years and much lower than the average of 71 years in the developed world. The population per physician, which averaged 5,208 between 1990 and 1999 further reinforces the precarious position of the Nigerian health system (Table 7.2).

Public expenditure on health was only 0.7 per cent of GDP for the period between 1990 and 1997. This probably accounts for the country's poor health outcomes as exemplified in a high maternal mortality rate, which was almost 36 per cent higher than the African average in 1999. It could also account for the level of crude death rate, which is slightly higher than the African average.

50

Table 7.2: Comparative Health and Social Indicators, Nigeria

Indicator	Year	Nigeria	Africa
GNI per Capita (US$)	2000	260	671
Labour Force Participation Total (million)	2000	50.3	290.5
Life Expectancy at Birth (years)	1999	46	51
Infant Mortality Rate (per 1000)	1999	83	87
Maternal Mortality Rate (per 100,000 live births)	1999	1,000	734
Total Fertility Rate (Birth per woman)	2000	5.2	4.9
Crude Birth Rate (per 1000 live births)	1999	39.8	37.2
Crude Death Rate (per 1000 of the population)	1999	15.7	14.5
Population per Physician	1990-'99	5,208	Na
Population per Hospital Bed	1990-'98	599	1,133
Access to Safe Water (%)	1990-'98	49	56
Access to Sanitation Facilities (%)	1995-2000	63	60
Percentage of births attended by trained health Personnel	1990-'99	26	43.7
Daily Calorie per Capita	1992	2,147	2,335
Public Expenditure on Health (% of GDP)	1990-'97	0.7	2.2

Source: African Development Indicators, 2002
World Development Indicators, 2002

Though access to sanitation facilities in Nigeria is above the African average, only 49 per cent of the population has access to safe water, lower than the African average of 56 per cent. Shortage of health personnel in the country is epitomized by the low percentage of births attended by trained personnel, which was only 26 per cent in the 1990s, much below the African average of 43.7 per cent.

7.4 Burden of Diseases

Infectious diseases characterize the Nigerian epidemiological pattern. This has been worsened by malnutrition and high fertility in recent times. The Nigerian epidemiological environment is dominated by the prevalence of malaria, infecting 919 per 100,000. This problem is further aggravated by the existence of drug-resistant malaria. The occurrence of resistance to malaria drugs increased from 2 per cent in 1992 to 40 per cent in 1996, while a variation in resistance to malaria by location in the country ranged between 20 per cent and 50 per cent in 1999 (Olumese, 1999). Other common diseases like dysentery which has a prevalence rate of 386 per 100,000 people; pneumonia, 146 per 100,000 and measles, 89 per 100,000 people (FMOH, 2000).

The World Bank (1994a) also noted that Nigeria is characterized by such other endemic diseases like dracunculiasis, schistosomiasis and onchocerciasis, with

51

associated illness burden and loss of economic productivity. Other water-borne diseases like diarrhea and typhoid are also becoming diseases of serious public health concern due to the breakdown of infrastructure throughout the country. Also diseases like cerebrospinal meningitis (CSM), yellow fever and Lassa fever are occurring with increased frequency in epidemic proportion.

Diseases of the transition are also on the increase in Nigeria. Thus, FMOH (2000) asserted that there is a growing incidence of and prevalence of non-communicable diseases like hypertension, coronary heart diseases, diabetes, cancer and stress-related illness as well as behaviourally - and life-style-induced health risks and problems. The prevalence of hypertension is estimated at 8-10 per cent in rural areas and 10-12 per cent in urban communities, according to a survey of non-communicable diseases in the country in 1989. The proportion of smokers was estimated at 9 per cent while prevalence of diabetes mellitus was 2.75 per cent. Such genetic diseases like sickle cell and glucose-6-phosphate dehydrogenate also affect an appreciable proportion of the population. The prevalence of the latter was estimated at 18 per cent and 7 per cent respectively for males and females.

Though first reported in 1986, the incidence and burden of HIV/AIDS is on the increase in the country such that its doubt or denial is no longer possible. The prevalence rate estimated to be 1.8 per cent in 1993, increased by more than 100 per cent within a year to 3.8 per cent in 1994, then to 4.5 per cent in 1996 and 5.4 per cent in 1999 (Table7.3).

Table 7.3: Incidence of HIV/AIDS in Nigeria (1999)

People	Prevalence
Adults (15-49)	2,600,000
Adult Rate of Growth (%)	5.1
Women (15-49)	1,400,000
Children (0-14)	120,000
AIDS Death	250,000

Source: African Development Indicators, 2002

Table 7.3 shows that more than 2 million of the total population are infected by HIV/AIDS in Nigeria. It also shows that the number of women affected by HIV/AIDS is greater than that of men. The estimated death as a result of HIV/AIDS was also 250,000 in 1999, which is almost a quarter of the number of HIV/AIDS death recorded in Africa in 1999. There is zonal variation in the prevalence of the pandemic in the country with the North- central zone being the worst hit, having a prevalence of 8.6 per cent (Table 7.4).

Table 7.4: HIV/AIDS Prevalence by Zone in Nigeria (%)

Zone	Urban	Rural	Total
South-east	7.1	4.6	7.1
South-west	4.7	2.9	4.1
South-south	5.4	6.4	6.1
North-west	5.8	3.0	3.8
North-east	4.5	4.8	3.5
North-central	8.2	8.7	8.6
Nigeria			5.4

Source: *FMOH (2000)*

Urban centres also tend to be more prone to HIV /AIDS infection than rural areas in most zones except in the North-central and South-south zones where prevalence is higher in rural areas.

7.5   Health Institutional Setup, Policies, Plans and Programmes

The thrust of the National Health Policy (NPH), adopted in 1988, with the objective of providing health for all Nigerians, is the improvement of Primary Health Care (PHC) programmes. The NPH places emphasis, as part of its implementation on the provision of comprehensive maternal and child health (MCH) services, including the family planning services, at the community level as part of PHC. It also places strong linkage between the PHC and Secondary Health Care (SCH) facilities through referral services. In fact, the SCH facilities serve as the apex of health care delivery for PHC in each of the 774 Local Government Areas (LGAs) in the country. Accordingly, each LGA is expected to have at least one functional and well-equipped SCH facility to enhance health care delivery at this level.

The health system in Nigeria, is organized in a three-tiered pyramidal structure that is comprehensive in nature, multi-sectoral in inputs, collaborative in planning and implementation and employing the active participation of communities and NGOs (FMOH, 1988). At the base of this pyramid is the PHC consisting of a network of clinics, health posts, dispensaries, maternity centres, health centres and comprehensive health centres. The second level consists of the SHC facilities, which are made up of general and state hospitals. Specialist and teaching hospitals constitute the third tiers- the tertiary health care level.

The three governmental tiers in Nigeria approximate the supervision, control and responsibility for the three levels of health care delivery. The PHC, is in general, mainly taken care of by local governments, while the SCH facilities are mainly the responsibilities of state governments and that of the Federal Government, is in the main, responsible for tertiary health care. The Federal Ministry of Health (FMOH) has overall responsibility for the health sector in terms of setting policies and providing guidelines to the states and the Federal Capital Territory. Besides, it has direct operational responsibility for the following:

- Coordination of state effort towards a nation-wide health system;
- Monitoring and evaluation of the implementation of national health strategy;
- Training of doctors;
- Setting uniform standards for all health workers;
- Operating institutions and services that are of national character like teaching, psychiatric and orthopaedic hospitals;
- Control of communicable diseases; and
- Supplies of vaccines and seed money for drug funds.

The FMOH also maintains a formal linkage with the different states through the National Council of Health consisting of all State Commissioners for Health, which is chaired by the Federal Minister of Health.

At the state level, the State Ministry of Health (SMOH) takes charge of the health care and is assisted by the State Hospitals Management Board (SHMB), which is responsible for the operations of state secondary health care facilities. The political head of the SMOH is the State Commissioner for Health who is responsible to the State Executive Council and is assisted by the Permanent Secretary of the SMOH as technical and administrative head. Among the main functions of the SMOH are:

- Planning the development of the health system of the state;
- Overseeing the operation and maintenance of secondary and non-tertiary specialized hospitals such as general, state and district hospitals;
- Implementing public health programmes;
- Training nursing, midwifery, and auxiliary health personnel; and assisting LGAs to manage their network of PHC facilities; and
- Determining the policies and guidelines through the SHMB functions and maintaining overall responsibility for the state's health programmes.

Each of the 774 LGAs in Nigeria has overall responsibility for PHC in its area of jurisdiction, including community health activities such as immunization and health education; hygiene and sanitation services; and provision of basic outpatient services at its maternity centres, clinics, dispensaries and health posts. Of course, states provide supportive linkage to LGAs through management of referrals from the PHC level to the SCH level as well as technical guidance (ADB,1992).

54

The NHP was the first major policy document on health in Nigeria. Its main innovation relates to explicitly making PHC the corner stone of health care delivery throughout the country as advocated by the Alma Ata Conference of 1978. Additionally, it emphasizes the availability of adequate referral support for PHC-oriented services through the rehabilitation of SHC facilities, which are required in each LGA to serve as an apex for PHC provision. The development of NPH opened the floodgates for a number of other policy documents focusing on specific health sector issues or crosscutting issues affecting the sector and others. Thus, there are policy documents addressing specific issues and subject areas like disease control, malaria, and child health, HIV/AIDS, for example or overall sector issue like health sector reforms; health management information system; and crosscutting issues like population and nutrition. It is instructive that while these documents focus on different issues relating to the health sector or its sub-sectors, the NPH, in general, provides the basic fulcrum.

More recently, the vision of the health sector and the direction in which it plans to steer in the foreseeable future are depicted in a number of policy documents like *Health Sector Reform Strategic Health Plan and Plan of Action*, 2000-2002 (October, 1999). Others are *Health System Development Project (HSDP) Implementation Plan* (August 2000); and *Health Sector Reform Medium Term Plan of Action 2001-2003*. All these policy documents are related. The Health Sector Reform (HSR), Strategic Plan and Plan of Action and the HSR Medium Term Plan Action are derived from NHP, the draft National Health Plan, the National Vision 2010 Report including President Obasanjo's health priority statements as well as varied consultative inputs from across the country. The consultative process aims at ensuring consensus building. This process brought together State Governors, Ministers, senior policy-level staff from the FMOH, State Honourable Commissioners for Health, LGA Chairmen and their Supervisory Counselors for Health, Heads of Departments of Health in the LGAs, representatives of tertiary health care institutions and the organized private sector, NGOs and members of the press.

The Medium Term Plan of Action distilled twelve broad objectives, which are planned to be achieved during the period 2001-2003. These cover such areas as primary health care (1 objective); disease control (2 objectives); sexual and reproductive health including STD/HIV/AIDS (1 objective); secondary and tertiary care (2 objectives); drug production and management (2 objectives); co-ordination of development with partners (1 objective); and organization and management (3 objectives). For each objective or group of objectives, the Plan of Action sets out outputs/targets as well as indicators of evaluation. The plan provides a logical framework summary of the required output for each objective/group of objectives as well as the outline of activities to achieve the output. It also provides the framework for the institutions to carry out the activities, the agencies whose support is crucial to the achievement of the objectives/output and the estimated costs.

The HSDP Project Implementation Plan is a follow-up to the Health System Fund (HSF) Project financed by the World Bank through the Nigeria Technical Co-operation Agreement. The agreement provides for the mobilization and utilization of development assistance including access to soft IDA-type facilities to complement national resources to finance national development, planning and programming. The HSDP derives its guiding principles and strategies from the strategic vision of the HSR objectives. Because of resource limitations, it focuses on interventions in areas it considers of highest priority to achieve maximum impact. Its four areas of strategic focus are:

- Strengthening health services (including PHC and referral services, in terms of drugs, infrastructure, facilities, and community involvement);
- Strengthening disease control (specifically in the areas of vaccine-preventable diseases, maternal and reproductive health, including HIV/AIDS;
- Improving the performance of the health system (specifically through health human resource development, technical assistance in system development); and
- Strengthening evidence, health statistics and information base for health system performance assessment and policy.

The other policy documents in the area of HIV/AIDS control are of prime importance to ensuring the improved health status of Nigerians in the years to come. These are National Action Committee on AIDS (NACA), Interim Action Plan, and the Nigerian: HIV/AIDS Program Development Aide Memoire. The latter is an improvement on the former and will likely form the basis of the programme of action of NACA. Accordingly, it will be focused upon more. This document prioritized the activities of NACA to ensure effective AIDS control. Its activities can be put into three groups according to geographical coverage: national level activities; nation-wide state-and LGA-level activities; and activities to be carried out in eighteen states at the state and local government levels but in a phased manner. The plan lists considered by this document are implementation arrangements including roles and responsibilities; lines of accountability, financial and auditing arrangements and procurement issues; monitoring and evaluation as well as donor co-ordination.

Health system programmes and projects are undertaken at different levels. Two types of funding sources readily come to mind: they are domestic and foreign sources. At the domestic front, fund can come from government and the private sector. The private sector includes for profit or organized private sector; the civil society includes the community, NGOs and Missions. Foreign sources can be bilateral or multilateral agencies as well as NGOs. For this review, however, we will use two documents as our guide in order to gain an insight into what the situation looks like in Nigeria. The first is the HSDP and the second is the HIV/AIDS Programme Development Aide Memoir.

The HSDP proposes to execute two categories of projects each covering the four priority areas described earlier. The two classes are: State Health sub-projects, which covers strengthening health services; strengthening maternal and child health services including reproductive health, and building and strengthening the health system institutional capacity. Others are strengthening the health management information system; and FMOH component of HSDP consisting of strengthening the National Health Management Information System (NHMIS), building and strengthening the health system institutional capacity, as well as HSDP project co-ordination.

The national level projects (states and the federal) plan to spend a total of $275,787,775 out of which $27,998,269 will be counterpart fund. Strengthening health care delivery (primary, secondary and tertiary care) will take the lion's share of $169,228,392 or 61.4%, while improvement in maternal and child health including reproductive health will consume $18,289,993(6.6%). Institutional capacity building will take $73,808,715(26.8%) and establishment of health management information system is expected to cost $14,460,735(5.2%).

The Interim Action Plan and the Aide Memoire for HIV/AIDS proposes projects based on eight strategies namely: promotion of behaviour change, generating and using technical information, ensuring adequate resources, and developing institutional capacity. It also includes targeting interventions, for general population, and care and support for persons affected by HIV/AIDS. These activities and project can be grouped into three categories: prevention activities, care and support. A total of $182,100,501 is estimated for the plan of which Nigeria is expected to provide nearly 30% while development partners like the UK Department for International Development (DFID), Centre for Disease Control (CDC) in the US, International Development Administration (IDA), the United States Agency for International Development (USAID), the United Nations Children's Fund (UNICEF), the US Departments of Labour and Defense, the World Health Organization (WHO) and others, will provide the balance.

PART THREE

POST-CONFLICT HEALTH CARE IN CONFLICT COUNTRIES

Chapter Eight

ASSESSING POST-CONFLICT HEALTH CARE IN GUINEA-BISSAU

8.1 Introduction

As stated earlier in this book, the study of the 'State of Post-Conflict Health Care Delivery in West Africa' aims at assessing the state of readiness of West African countries in addressing the problems of health care delivery under conflict with a view to developing a proactive approach at national and regional levels for solving the ensuing problems. Guinea-Bissau was selected as one of the countries that had witnessed one or more conflicts in the past. A number of visits were conducted to collect data for the study. The first visit, which was conducted in October 2001 appointed the country coordinator and briefed the research team, which was raised earlier on the four sets of survey instruments being used for the study to solicit information from the Ministry of Public Health, health facilities, NGOs and policy makers on various issues of post-conflict health care in the country. The visit was also used to assess various places, which had been destroyed during the civil war, and to conduct some informal interviews with some of the peacekeeping personnel as well as some of the nationals. The second visit, which took place in the first quarter of 2002 was used to retrieve the completed questionnaires.

8.2 The Country: Guinea-Bissau and the Role of Government

Guinea-Bissau is a relatively small country. Most of its land area is swampy and under water. Accordingly, many of the villages and communities are inaccessible. The civil war made its health system suffer various inadequacies particularly in regard to health facilities, personnel, funding and supplies, among others. All the major buildings like the presidential villa, the Central Bank, and other public buildings were all destroyed.

The country also has a very high level of poverty. The physical structures of the major urban centres like Bissau, Jeta, Biombo and Gabu confirm this assertion on the level of poverty in the country. It also lacks basic infrastructural facilities like good roads, electricity supply and telecommunications. In fact, there is no road network that links the country with its neighbours such as Senegal and the Republic of Guinea. This is apart from the fact that the devastating effects of the civil war compounded this already precarious poverty problem with the destruction of the country's limited facilities.

The high infant and maternal mortality rates in various rural and urban hospitals in the country bear clear attestation to the deplorable state of the country's health system. As shown earlier, the country's infant mortality rate in 1999 was 127 per 1,000 live births while the corresponding maternal mortality rate was 910 per 100,000 live births. With a physician attending, on average to 5,665 persons between 1990 and 1999; and with a population/bed ratio of 677 between 1990 and 1998, the observed poor outcomes of the health system of Guinea-Bissau, will be seen to be the results of shortages of critical inputs into the health system like physicians and hospital beds, among others. The high shortage of skilled manpower in the country's health system, is also, in part, a reflection of the absence of tertiary and other professional institutions like a university for building such high human capital capacity in the country. Thus, all the country's university graduates are products of foreign institutions in Guinea, Senegal, France and Portugal, while the country's official language is Portuguese.

Communicable diseases constitute the highest source of morbidity in Guinea-Bissau. The high incidence and burden of diseases like diarrhea, tuberculosis and malaria attest to the poor nature of the PHC facilities in the country. The incidence and burden of HIV/AIDS became worse during and after the civil war. The presence of peacekeeping personnel really increased the level of prostitution in the country. With the destruction of the Sheraton Hotel in Bissau, one of the remaining major hotels in the country, the '24 Septembro', accommodated and kept the majority of the peacekeeping personnel, providing an avenue for the influx of young girls and ladies involved in prostitution. This may, in part, account for the increase in HIV/AIDS patients in the hospitals. This is in agreement with the literature of post-conflict health care which asserts that one of the indirect effects of conflict on the health system is the possible increase in the levels of prostitution, which may occur as female heads of households seek cash income in the absence of other productive activities. In addition, the breakdown in the health services would lead to reduced opportunities for treating STDs which may increase the vulnerability of conflict-affected communities to HIV infection (Zwi, and Cabral, 1991; Smallman-Raynor and Cliff, 1991; Bond and Vincent, 1990 and Macrae, Zwi and Forsythe, 1995b). It is not surprising, therefore that of the 15 – 49 year-old adults estimated to have HIV/AIDS in the country in 1999, 7,300 or 56% are women. As many as 1,300 persons are estimated to have died of AIDS in the country while the disease orphaned 6,100 children in 1999.

In Guinea-Bissau, health care delivery at the three primary, secondary and tertiary levels of care, is provided at national, regional and district hospitals, as well as health centres and community-managed village health posts (USBs). There are two national hospitals, four regional hospitals, twelve district hospitals, 121 health centres and 450 village health posts in the entire country.

The Ministry of Public Health (MINSAP) oversees the provision of health services at national and other levels. Our survey revealed that the country has no formal policy or guidelines for addressing issues relating to post-conflict health care. However, it relies on the 1976 Health Plan and various interventions of international organizations like UNICEF, UNDP and the WHO to finance and address issues that may crop up in this connection. The 1976 Health Plan emphasizes decentralization of services, preventive care (without neglecting curative care) and the use of simple techniques and practices as well as the training of all personnel including volunteer staff like village health workers and village midwives.

In terms of personnel, the country suffers from a dearth of qualified personnel, particularly with the effects of the civil war. Many of the health centres are without nurses, not to talk of doctors. The village health posts (USBs) are based on community-participation with a significant amount of local-resource mobilization and sharing of responsibility between community leaders/members in the villages and the MINSAP defined by contract letters between the relevant parties. However, the effective performance of the system is highly constrained by the high level of poverty of the citizenry in spite of their high level of enthusiasm.

The effects of the civil war tend to tell adversely on the many assets of MINSAP. This is vividly captured by looking at some of its buildings like that of the *Hospital Nacional Simao Mendes*, part of which was razed while the remaining parts which were partially destroyed were used by all departments of MINSAP as at the time of our survey. As if to compound the problem resulting from the shortage of accommodation for MINSAP, part of the building complex of the ministry was taken over as one of the official residences of the Head of State (Figure 8.1). This can be seen as compounding the problem of asset shortages for post-conflict health care in the country, even at the highest administrative level. It is not out of place, therefore, to conjecture, even at this early stage of the study that the corresponding problem at the lower level of health care delivery in the country, particularly at the facility level, can better be imagined.

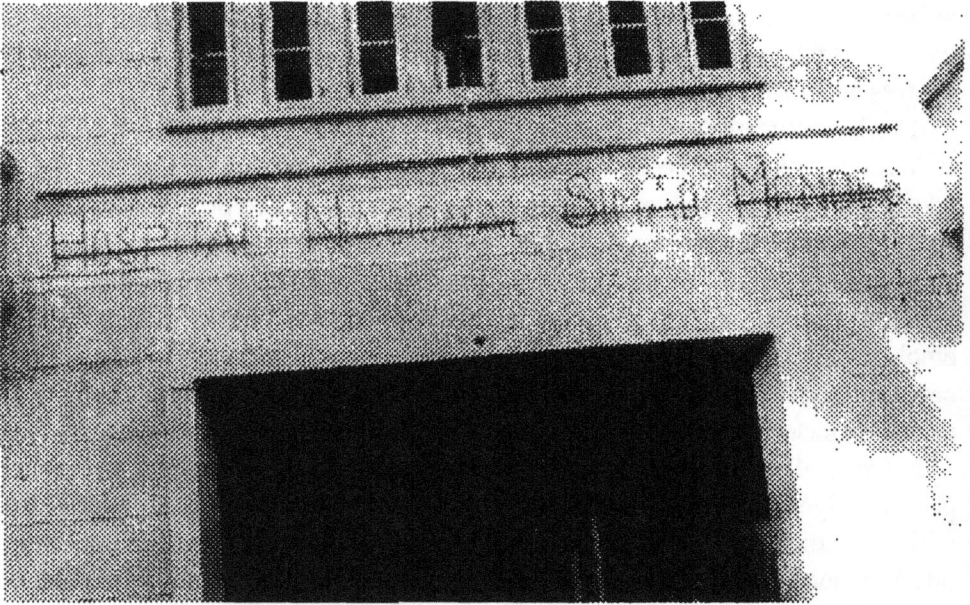

Picture 8.1: *Part of the MINSAP Building Complex Used as One of the Head of State's Official Residences*

The *Hospital de Agosto* in Bissau that was used for treating patients with infectious diseases was also destroyed during the civil war (Figure 8.2). This mounted a lot of pressure on the General Hospital in the city. This adverse effect on the hospital stretched the already inadequate facilities of the General Hospital to their limit, leading to increasing mortality. Besides, an annex to the building, which served as a children's ward, was also destroyed (Figure 8.3). The subsequent effect of this destruction was the pressure that was put on the Catholic Hospital in Bissau. Luckily, this hospital was not touched during the civil war and it served as an important treatment centre for the country during and after the war.

One of the major laboratories in the country, the LNSP, was also partially destroyed during the civil war. At the time of our field visit, it was undergoing refurbishment. The effect of this event was the high cost incurred by patients in carrying out laboratory tests. However, interventions by such agencies as UNICEF, WHO and the *Catholica Nationale* which carried out tests for some patients at minimal or no costs at all helped in ameliorating the ensuing problems (Figure 8.4).

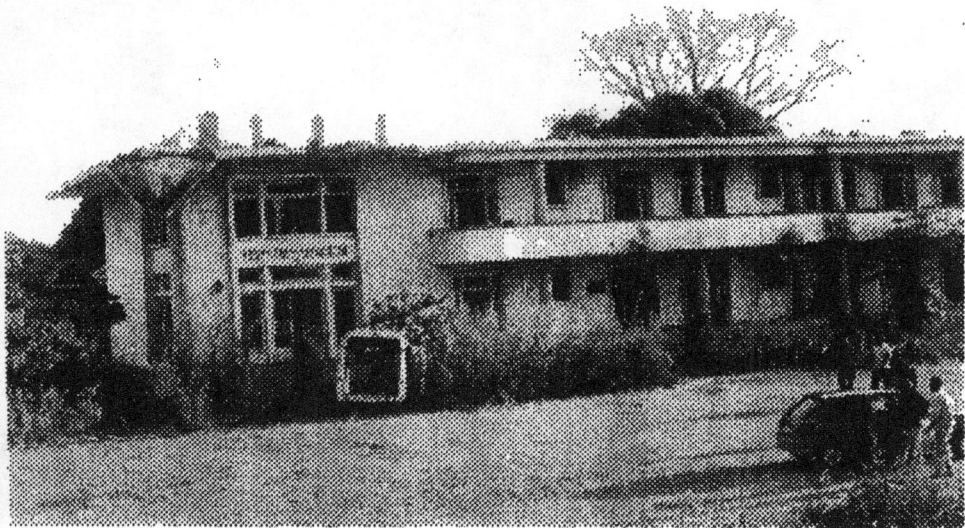

Picture 8.2: *Part of the Hospital de Agosto in Bissau Destroyed During the War*

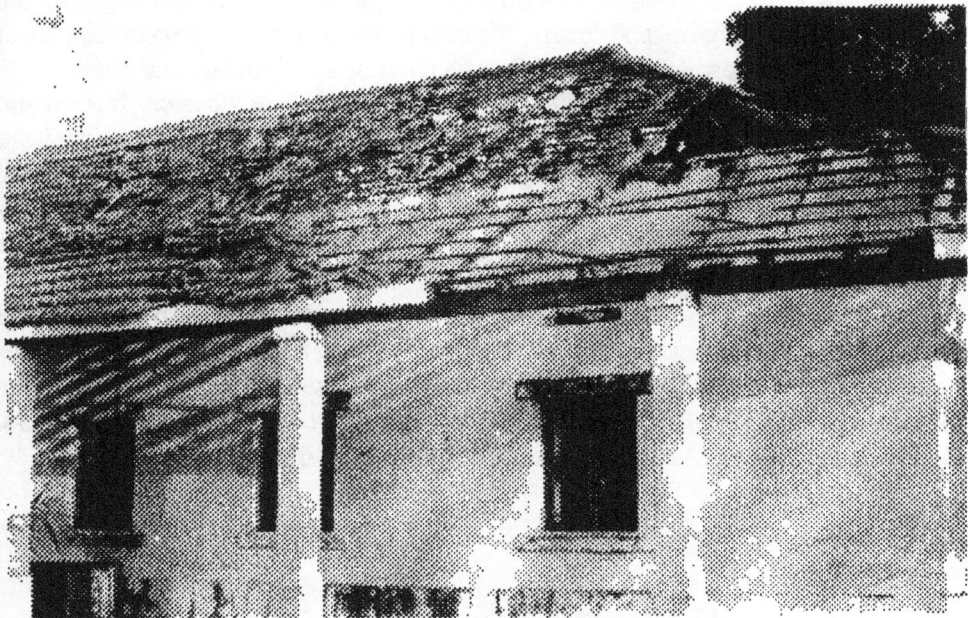

Picture 8.3: *Annex of the General Hospital for Children Health Services*

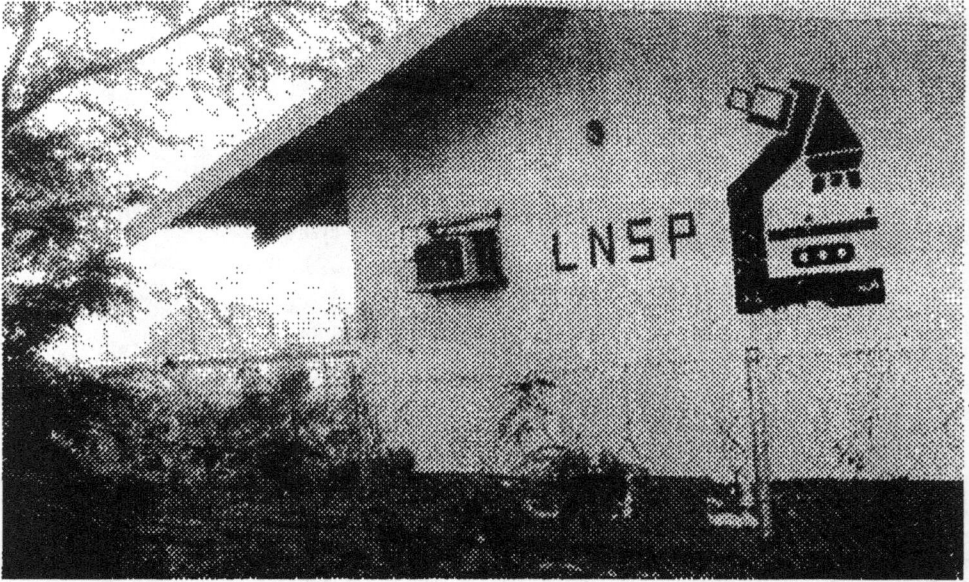

Picture 8.4: *LNSP, One of the Major Laboratories in the Country Which Was Badly Affected by the War* **(Effect of Destruction in the Background)**

The General Hospital in Bissau also had a taste of the destruction resulting from the civil war. Being a large establishment, the effects of the destruction were felt only in some parts of the hospital (Figures 8.5 and 8.6). In spite of the fact that even before the civil war, the country lacked the necessary infrastructure, physical; human and policy/legislative; the civil war aggravated the situation, thereby destroying a significant part of the limited assets of the health system of Guinea-Bissau. Bissau, the capital was terribly hit by the civil war. The national, regional and district hospitals as well as the health centres and village health posts, were ill-equipped to accommodate the influx of people into the rural areas, a situation created by the civil war in the country. In fact, the lack of good roads and the problems posed by the war made the rural areas inaccessible for health workers, thereby recording high death rates in refugees who otherwise might have received treatment. These findings corroborate the assertions of the literature of the health system under conflict like Luxen (1997), Macrae (1997), and Macrae, Zwi and Forsythe (1995b).

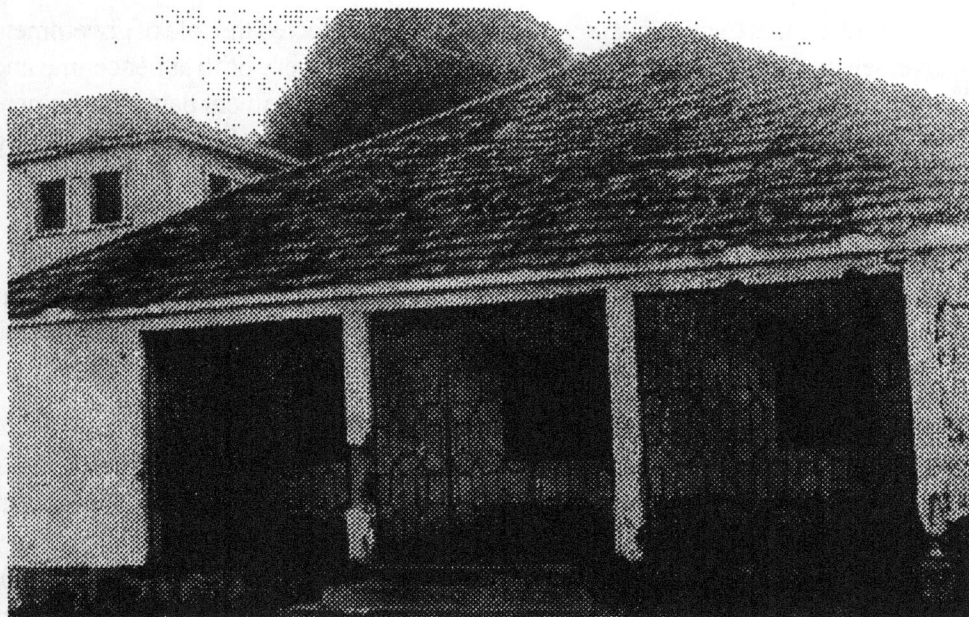

Picture 8.5: *A Part of the General Hospital Destroyed During the War*

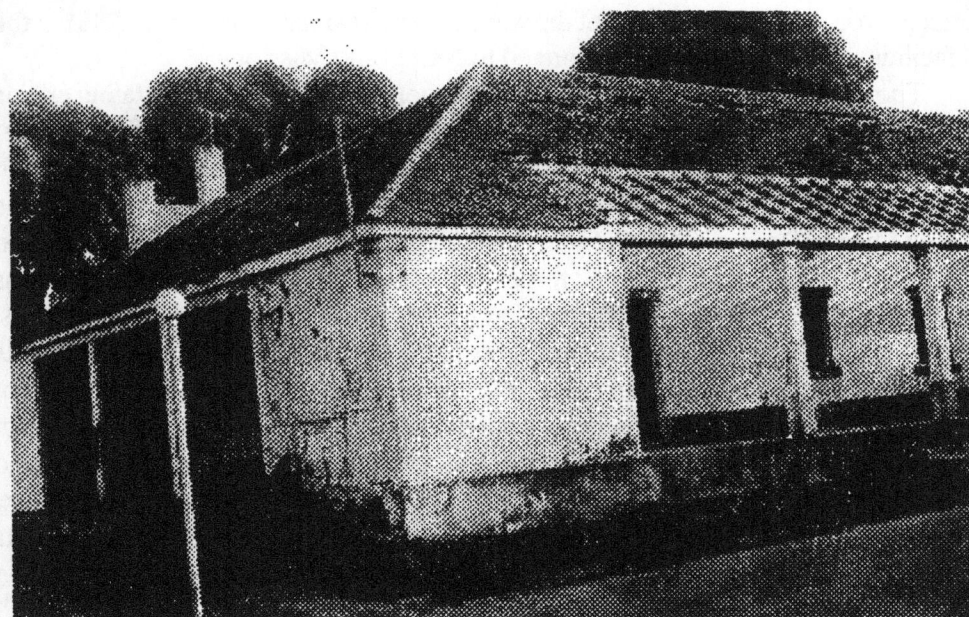

Picture 8.6: *Effect of the War on Another Part of the General Hospital*

This suggests that the ensuing poverty in the country affected the role of government adversely in contributing effectively to health care delivery both at peacetime and under conflict. As will be seen later, largely those of development partners augment the contribution of government to the budgets of the health facilities both during peacetime and under situations of conflict.

8.3   Impact of Conflicts on Health Care Facilities

We analyze the effects of conflicts on sampled health care facilities of Guinea-Bissau. This is expected to reveal particular characteristics of the facilities and the extent of the impact of the war on them, including their assets and personnel.

8.3.1   Characteristics of Respondent Facilities

A total of 28 facilities were surveyed in Guinea Bissau. The majority of the facilities that were surveyed, 20 or 71.4% were owned by the for-profit private sector. The Government owned only 6 or 21.4%. Hospitals in the tertiary/secondary level of health care delivery constituted the majority of the sample (15 or 53.6%). Of these, 14 or 50% were owned by the for-profit private sector. Health facilities at the primary care level that were surveyed were 13 or 46.4%. Over 82% of the facilities surveyed were in the urban areas. This is justified by our review earlier in this chapter where it was indicated that it was difficult for people to access health care in the rural areas during the war because of the twin problems of lack of good access roads and the intensity of the war in the rural areas. Only two (7.2%) of the facilities that were surveyed belonged to NGOs and Missions.

Though the conflict in Guinea-Bissau is reported to have had devastating effects on the health system of the country, it did not last for too long. All the facilities that were surveyed indicated that it lasted between 1998 and 1999. The conflict began with a rebellion in June 1998 by units of the armed forces of the country led by the then Chief of Defence Staff. President Joao Bernardo Vieira of Guinea-Bissau asked for the intervention of the armed forces of the Republics of Guinea and Senegal as indicated by ECOWAS (2000) on account of the bilateral and security agreements. Also, at the request of the lawful authority in the country and in order to reaffirm its support for the elected government of Guinea-Bissau, the ECOWAS Authority of Heads of States and Governments decided to restore peace and reinstate President Vieira in authority over the entire country. A mechanism for the supervision and control of cease-fire was set up by ECOWAS with contingents of soldiers sent in by Benin, Niger and Togo. However, in spite of the numerous cease-fire agreements signed by the parties in the conflict in Guinea-Bissau, the democratically elected government of Guinea-Bissau was overthrown leading to the civil war.

8.3.2 Effects of Conflict on Human and Other Resources and Service Operations

(A) Human Resources

The conflict in Guinea-Bissau had differing impacts on the different health personnel categories. Before the conflict, there were on the average, 2.30 doctors in each of the surveyed facilities. This decreased by 50.4% to 1.14 per facility during the first year of the conflict, dropping marginally by about 10% to 1.03 per facility during the second year of the conflict Table 8.1. The effect on the number of nurses was not as acute as on the number of doctors. Thus, before the conflict, there were on average 3.69 nurses in each of the facilities surveyed. This dropped by about 4% to 3.55 per facility during the first year of the conflict and further by 12.3% to 3.11 per facility during the second year of the conflict. The impact of the civil war on the supply of pharmacists in the country's health facilities is much worse than that on nurses but not as bad as the impact on the supply of doctors. Before conflict, for example, the average number of pharmacists in each of the surveyed facilities was 2.18. This dropped sharply by 31.2% to 1.50 per facility during the first year of the war, dropping further by 22% to 1.17 per facility during the second year of the conflict. The supply of other health professionals was also adversely affected by the civil war in Guinea-Bissau.

On average, there were 3.27 other health professionals in each of the facilities surveyed before the conflict. This dropped by about 8% to 4.10 per facility during the first year of the conflict and further by 4% to 2.89 per facility during the second year of the conflict. For non-health professionals the story was almost virtually the same. There was a decrease between the average number of workers per facility between the year preceding the war and the first year of the conflict. This was 4.30 per facility before the conflict, dropping by about 5% to 4.10 per facility during the first year of the conflict. However, it increased by more than 3.46 times to 18.3 per facility during the second year of the conflict.

The results of our survey on the average number of health facility staff in Guinea-Bissau, while generally below the norm as found by Eklund and Staven (1996), however, contrast with some of their findings. For example, they found that on average, there were 1.3 doctors per facility; our survey indicated some improvement of 2.30 before the conflict and worse performance during the first and second years of the conflict. However, all the results were below the norm of 2.7 per facility. For nurses, Eklund and Staven (1996) found that on average, health facilities of Guinea-Bissau had 1.3 per facility. In contrast, our survey found an average of 3.69 per facility before the conflict and 3.55 during the first year of the conflict and 3.11 during the second year of the conflict. The norm is 5.3 per facility. Thus, there is no gaining the fact that the health system of Guinea-Bissau is bedeviled by serious personnel shortages even in peacetime. The results also corroborate the observations of Luxen (1997), Macrae, Zwi, and

69

Forsythe (1995a&b) Macrae (1997) on the impact of conflict on the human resources of the health system.

Table 8.1: Effects of Conflict on Staff (Average Number)*

Variable	Before Conflict	Year 1 of Conflict	Year 2 of Conflict	Year 1 After Conflict	Year 2 After Conflict
Number of doctors	2.30	1.14	1.03	1.40	2.08
Number of nurses	3.69	3.55	3.11	3.94	3.86
Pharmacists	2.18	1.50.	1.17	1.50	1.93
Other Health professional staff	3.27	3.01	2.89	3.00	3.00
Non-health professional staff	4.30	4.10	18.3	4.89	35.90

* Rounding-off not done so as not to mask the effects of conflict, however marginal.

The literature of health care under conflict, asserts that post-conflict situations tend to improve the supply of health personnel. Thus, the average number of doctors improved from 1.40 per facility a year after the conflict by 48.6% to 2.08 in the second year after the conflict. The supply of nurses in health facilities showed an improvement of 26.7% between the first year after the conflict and the second year of conflict. However, it experienced a slight decline of 2.0% between the first and second years after the conflict. The average number of pharmacists per facility also improved with the advent of peace. Thus on average, there were 1.50 pharmacists per facility during the first year after the conflict. This increased by 28.7% to 1.93 during the second year after the conflict. While the average number of other health professionals increased marginally (3.8%) between the second year of the conflict and the first year after the conflict, there was no change in the value between the first and second years after the conflict. It is with the supply of non-health professional staff that an impact of peace appears most dramatic, in Guinea-Bissau. The average number of staff per facility increased by more than six times between the first and second years after the conflict! Under post-conflict situations, in spite of some improvements over conflict situations, Guinea-Bissau is still beset by shortages. Comparing with the norm specified by Eklund and Staven (1996), the average number of doctors per facility standing at 1.40 and 2.08 during the first and second years after the conflict respectively is below the norm of 2.7. Similarly, the average number of nurses per facility of 3.94 a year after the conflict and 3.86 during the second year after the conflict fell short of the norm of 5.3 per facility.

70

Table 8.2: Effects of Conflict on Other Resources and the Management Process: Guinea-Bissau(Average Number/Amount)

Variable	Before Conflict	Year1 of Conflict	Year 2 of Conflict	Year 1 After Conflict	Year After Conflict
Number of Management meetings	1.58	0.58	0.02	6.50	2.29
Number of staff sent on training	14.33	0.01	-	3.80	1.00
Number of out-patients	556.0	985 .71	2046.8	490.75	452.0
Number of in-patients	12.67	452.78	-	115.00	-
Number of wards	10.25	10.25	9.32	11.67	12.88
Number of functioning wards	8.87	6.77	5.64	11.67	12.54
Approved budget (Million Pesos)	5.84	4.50	1.08	5.90	4.07
Actual expenditure (Million Pesos)	12.88	12.00	6.00	12.00	2.98

(B) Other Resources

While there was no change in the average number of wards per facility between the year before the conflict and the first year of the conflict, there was a decline of 9.1% from 10.25 to 9.32 between the first and second years of the conflict. In Guinea-Bissau, the conflict appeared to have more of an impact on the availability of functioning wards. The average number of functioning wards declined from 8.87 per facility before the conflict to 6.77 by 23.7% during the first year of the conflict (Table 8.2). This further declined by 16.7% to 4.64 in the second year of the conflict. The decrease in the average number of functioning wards will be seen to be multiples of the average number of wards available. This is in agreement with Macrae, Zwi and Forsythe (1995); Luxen (1997); Macrae (1997) on the effects of conflict on the health infrastructure. The cessation of hostilities had a lot of positive effects on health infrastructure of Guinea-Bissau. Between the second year of the conflict and the first year after the conflict, the average number of functioning wards increased 106.9% from 5.64 to 11.67. This further increased to 12.54 by 14.1% during the second year after the conflict.

In general, in Guinea-Bissau, the actual expenditure per facility tends to be higher than the budget (except in the second year of conflict and the second year after conflict) suggesting that health facilities depended a lot on external assistance in funding their activities. Before the hostilities, the budget per facility was on average of the order 5.8 million pesos and this dropped by nearly 23% to 4.5 million pesos during the first year of conflict. Actual expenditure, which was, on average, 12.9 million pesos was 122.4% of the budget before the conflict. While the actual expenditure dropped to 12.0 million pesos by nearly 7% during the first year of the conflict, it was 166.7% of the budget for the year, suggesting that during the first year of the conflict, activities of health facilities in the country were financed more from non-governmental sources. The budget for during the second year conflict rose dramatically by 140% to 10.8 million pesos per facility during the second year of the conflict. However, this was the one of the two years in which our survey indicated that actual expenditure was less than the budget. The actual expenditure of 6.0 million pesos per facility was 55.6% of the budget. During the first year after the conflict, budget per facility dropped dramatically by 50% per facility to 5.9 million pesos while the actual expenditure increased by 50% to 12.0 million pesos suggesting the contribution of other partners and stakeholders to such a huge lift in budget performance of more than 103% actual/budget ratio. It will be recalled that earlier in this chapter, it was mentioned that the intervention of agencies like UNICEF and WHO helped in reducing the high cost of treatment to patients in the country, particularly with the devastating effects of war on the assets of the health system. Besides, the foregoing corroborates the assertions of Macrae, Zwi and Forsythe (1995b) that one of the major effects of conflict on the health system is the greater dependence of system financing on external aid.

(C) Management Processes and Service Operations

Conflict had deleterious effects on the management processes and operation of health services of the facilities surveyed. For example, before the conflict, on average, the facilities that were surveyed reported having 1.58 management meetings. However, during the first year of the conflict, this dropped by 63.3% to 0.58 and still further by nearly 97% to 0.02 during the second year of the conflict.[1] The training of staff appeared to suffer a lot from the effect of the conflict in Guinea-Bissau. On average, 14.33 staff per facility attended training per year before the conflict. This dropped by several multiples to 0.01 during the first year of conflict. In fact during the second year of the conflict none of the staff of all the facilities surveyed attended any training.

Under post-conflict situations, the conditions improved. Thus, the average number of management meetings went up to 6.50 during the first year after the conflict from 0.02 during the second year of the conflict, but declined by 64.8% to 2.29, during the second year after the conflict. The average number of staff attending training per facility also improved from nothing during the second year of the conflict to 3.80 per facility during the first year after the conflict. However, it declined by 73.7% to 1.00 during the second year after the conflict.

It appears that conflict increases the number of patients attending health facilities in Guinea-Bissau. Thus, the average number of out-patients increased from 556.0 during the year preceding the conflict by 77.3% to 985.71 during the first year of the conflict.[2] However, during the second year of the conflict, the average number of out-patients ballooned by nearly 107.7% to 2046.8 per facility. This finding is in agreement with literature of health delivery under conflict which asserts that health resources are diverted to treat more pressing war-related conditions in situations of conflict.

Nearly 25% of the facilities surveyed indicated that they were shut completely at one time other than during the time of hostilities. This contrasts sharply with the situation in Sierra Leone or Liberia as will be seen in Chapters Nine and Ten. It is not surprising that only a small proportion of the facilities in the country were closed because of conflict, given the fact that the conflict in Guinea-Bissau lasted for a short time of slightly more than a year. In contrast, both the conflict in Sierra Leone and Liberia lasted for a long time. Even at the time of writing, the conflict has only ceased (hopefully, completely) for about a year in Sierra Leone while in Liberia, a new band of rebels, at war with President Charles Taylor, were at the outskirts of Monrovia, and cease-fire negotiations were in progress in Accra, Ghana. Out of the 25% of the facilities that were closed, 17.9% were closed only once, 3.6% each were closed three times and four times (Figure 8.1). None was closed twice and assumed that the facilities under 'non-response' category (75.0%) were not closed at all.

Fig. 8.1: Conflict and Closure of Facilities: Guinea-Bissau

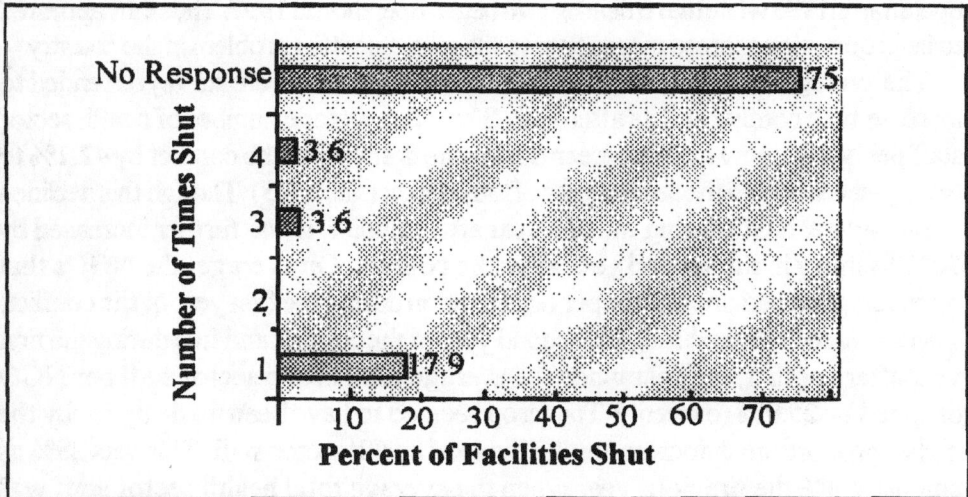

Some of the operators of facilities who were surveyed in Guinea-Bissau perceived that conflict had some negative effects on health care delivery in the country. Among the negative effects mentioned were:

73

- Leading to increased disability of staff and patients (46.4%);
- Causing shut-down of operations (42.9%);
- Causing migration of staff (35.7%);
- Causing destruction of equipment and facility (35.7%);
- Causing injury to patients and staff (25%);
- Increasing numbers of deaths of patients and staff (25%);
- Leading to increased cost of operation (14.3%); and
- Causing general dislocation of facilities.

Among the suggestions offered by the health facilities operators who were surveyed to improve the health care delivery while under conflict in Guinea-Bissau are:

- Enhancing drug provision;
- Providing health facilities in rural areas;
- Improving the conditions of workers;
- Increasing funding of health facilities by government and NGOs; and
- Ensuring that no organization exercises monopoly powers in training of health personnel.

8.4 The Roles of NGOs

For our analysis in this section, we shall use only three NGOs that returned usable, completed questionnaires. Of the three, only one is domestic and the other two are international. These NGOs began operations in the country quite recently. One began operation in 1996 while the remaining two began operation in 1997. Thus they appeared to be in operation moreso in response to the recent conflict problem in the country.

The average total health sector staff in the NGOs that were surveyed tended to increase with conflict and its aftermath. Thus, the average number of health sector staff per NGO, grew from nineteen during the first year of the conflict by 42.1% to twenty-seven during the second year of the conflict (Table 8.3). Though this declined to twenty per NGO during the first year after conflict, it was further increased by 50% to thirty in the second year after the conflict. On average, the NGOs that were surveyed had one doctor per organization during the first year of the conflict. This increased to two during the second year of the conflict and five during the first year after conflict, the year when the average total health sector staff per NGO dropped by 25.9% to twenty. This drop seemed to have been made up for by the higher proportion of doctors among the total health sector staff. This was 25% as against 7.4% the previous year when the average total health sector staff was twenty-seven per organization.

The average number of nurses per NGO was ten during the first and second years of the conflict. It dropped to 5.5 in the first year after the conflict when there was a dramatic increase in the proportion of doctors per NGOs. It would appear, there was a substitution of more doctors for nurses during the year by the NGOs surveyed. There was also a fall in the average number of non-health professional staff during the same year. Thus, in Guinea-Bissau, NGOs used more skilled professional inputs immediately after the cessation of hostilities, apparently because of complications resulting from the fresh impact of conflict. When the situation stabilized, like during the second year after the conflict they, then used personnel of less professional skill.

Table 8.3: NGO Health Personnel During and After Conflict:Guinea-
Bissau(Average Number)

Health Personnel	1st Year of Operation During Conflict	2nd Year of Operation During Conflict	1st Year After Conflict	2nd Year After Conflict
Doctors	1	2	5	2
Nurses	10	10	5.5	11
Pharmacists	-	-	1	1
Other Health Professional Staff	5	5	3	5
Non-health Professional Staff	10	10	5.5	11
Average Total Health Sector Staff	19	27	20	30

The NGOs that were surveyed perceived migration of their staff/loss of staff as the most important (100%) negative effect of conflict on their operations. Other negative effects identified were: destruction of health facilities/equipment; nonavailability or high cost of drugs; and increased health hazards and outbreak of epidemics.

They also identified problems and/or constraints to the effective delivery of health care under conflict situations in the country. These included:

- Lack of qualified or poor trained personnel;
- Poor logistics;
- Short supply or high cost of medication; and
- Lack of security.

Among the suggestions offered for ameliorating the identified problems were:

- Improvement in logistics;
- Increased funding by donors;
- Community mobilization/ restoration of local authorities; and
- Provision of less costly drugs.

It is not clear, given the situation on the ground that Guinea-Bissau has the capacity to coordinate the activities of NGOs effectively, particularly NGOs involved in health care delivery under conflict and in post-conflict situations. In particular, their activities appear restricted mainly to the short-term end of the relief-reconstruction and rehabilitation continuum. Clearly, their activities are not sustainable and the way they operate cannot assist in ensuring the containment of the critical rehabilitation dilemmas identified by Macrae (1997).

8.5 Health System Performance

The overall performance of the health system of Guinea-Bissau is captured by its ranking by the WHO *World Health Report* 2000 with an overall system ranking of 176 out of 191 countries. With this ranking, Guinea-Bissau ranks higher than both Liberia (181) and Sierra Leone (191). Using eight other measures, the performance of the health system of Guinea-Bissau is as follows:

- Health level(Disability-adjusted Life Expectancy – DALE): 170th;
- Health distribution: 177th;
- Responsiveness level: 184th;
- Responsiveness distribution: 174th;
- Fairness in financial contribution: 122nd - 123rd;
- Overall goal attainment: 180th;
- Health expenditure per capita in international dollars: 156th; and
- Performance on level of health: 156th.

Besides, UN(2002) also rates Guinea-Bissau alongside Liberia and Sierra Leone as belonging to the group of least developed nations of the world. It is also among the group of countries where a decline in fertility was yet to start by the year 2000. In particular, its total fertility during the period 1995-2000 was 6.99, better than both Sierra Leone and Liberia. Also, along with Liberia and Sierra Leone, Guinea-Bissau was listed by the document as being among twenty countries of the world with the lowest life expectancy, although its performance is relatively better than the other two study countries. Given the devastating effects of conflict on the health system and the people, the poor performance of the health system of Guinea-Bissau can, in part, be attributed to the conflict it recently experienced. In particular, its performance, which is relatively better than both Liberia and Sierra Leone, is likely to be due, in part, to relative shortness of the conflict experienced by the country.

8.6 Summary, Implications and Recommendations

The conflict in Guinea-Bissau, though relatively shorter than the ones in the two other study conflict countries, has some significant impacts on the health system and the population. One major effect is that, in spite of the limited availability of health infrastructure like buildings, one of the immediate effects of the conflict is that part of the

MINSAP building complex had to be appropriated as one of the official residences of the Head of State. Besides, the limited facilities like the General Hospital in Bissau, the *Hospital de Agosto* for treating infectious diseases, also in Bissau and LNSP, the major investigative laboratory in the country were destroyed as a result of the conflict.

MINSAP, the Ministry of Public Health oversees the provision of health services in the country. However, our study shows that the country has no formal policy or guidelines for addressing issues relating to post-conflict health care. Rather, it relies on the 1976 Health Plan and various interventions of international organizations like UNICEF, UNDP and the WHO to finance and address issues that may crop up in this connection. The 1976 Health Plan emphasizes decentralization of services, preventive care (without neglecting curative care) and the use of simple techniques and practices as well as the training of all personnel types including volunteer staff like village health workers and village midwives. More importantly, our study does not indicate whether the country has any coordinating agencies or policy or guidelines for monitoring NGOs operating in the country. This is particularly worrisome when it is realized that NGOs contributed a lot to health delivery under conflict in Guinea-Bissau. The effects will be that there will be possible duplication of efforts, wastages and redundancies in the activities of these organizations. Besides, the country will only take what the agencies provide rather than what it *needs*. Accordingly, health care delivery, under such a situation may not be sustainable, making the containment of the critical dilemmas of post-conflict health care (Macrae, 1997) difficult, if not impossible.

The conflict in Guinea-Bissau, though brief had significant effects on the supply of human resources in the health facilities surveyed. For example, the number of doctors per facility decreased from an average value of 2.30 before the conflict by 50.4% to 1.14 during the first year of conflict, thereafter dropping marginally by 10.1% to 1.03 during the second year of the conflict. Expectedly, during post-conflict situations, there was an improvement in the supply of health personnel to the facilities. The average number of doctors increased by 48.6% from 1.40 per facility during the first year after the conflict to 2.08 in the second year after the conflict. Others resources also suffered adversely from the effects of the conflict. The average number of functioning wards, for example, declined by 23.7% during the first year of the conflict. It declined further by 16.7% during the second year of the conflict. In contrast, cessation of hostilities improved the availability of functioning wards. The average number of functioning wards improved by 106.9% from 5.64 per facility to 11.67 between the second year of conflict and the first year after the conflict.

The conflict also had adverse effects on the management process in the facilities surveyed. The average number of management meetings, for example, decreased by 63.3% during the first year of the conflict and decreased further by nearly 97% during the second year of the conflict. Staff training, which appears to be a rare commodity in

77

the facility surveyed, suffered a drop of 99.94% during the first year of the conflict. Worse still, during the second year of the conflict, none of the facilities that were surveyed indicated sending any of their staff on training.

An important implication of this study is that Guinea-Bissau does not have the necessary institutional and legal framework to confront the problems of health care delivery in a sustainable way. Our study suggests that even the entire health system is operated, using a very old health plan, which does not seem to have been updated for a long time. With this scenario, it is difficult for the country to have developed institutional and legal framework to take care of specialized health care needs, as it is the case in health care delivery under conflict. It is important that the country develops the necessary framework for improving the performance of the entire health system in general and health care delivery under conflict, in particular. In this connection, the importance of creating a unit to coordinate the activities of NGOs and their contributions to health care delivery both during peacetime and under conflict cannot be overemphasized. This is with a view to ensuring that their activities and impact are sustainable in the long run and a duplication of efforts, wastages and redundancies are eliminated.

A major problem of the health system of Guinea-Bissau is not just the shortage of trained personnel, but also the non-availability of training institutions. There is no university in the country, hence its nationals are trained in Europe or neighbouring countries. As regards training for health care delivery under conflict, the problem is even more complex. Luckily, as will be seen later in this study, training programmes for capacity building in peace and conflict studies have begun in some universities in the West African subregion. This initiative and that to be provided by modifying the operation of existing regional health institutions can be adapted for training the required personnel, not only for Guinea-Bissau, but also for the entire West African subregion.

---

[1] This suggests that in Guinea-Bissau, holding of management meetings in health facilities appears not to be popular. This contradicts the guidelines of implementation of PHC where consultations among the various stakeholders including facility employees and the community, is strategic.

[2] The average numbers of out-patients and in-patients appear rather small that the figures look suspect. It may have something to do with the quality of record keeping at the facility level in the country.

Chapter Nine

ASSESSING POST-CONFLICT HEALTH CARE IN LIBERIA[1]

9.1 Introduction

Fieldwork in Liberia began with consultations with major stakeholders in post-conflict health care delivery in the country in late November 2001. The survey period covered November 2001 and the first quarter of 2002. For the survey of health facilities, a selection was done by purposive sampling based on prior knowledge from the country coordinator and his team of the different facilities, particularly in relation to the different services rendered, their areas of coverage and the length of time of operation in the country. A two-day training workshop was held for the enumerators engaged in the survey to familiarize them with the objectives of the study, its philosophy and the different instruments to be administered for data collection. '

One copy of each of Instruments 01 and 04 was administered on the Ministry of Health and Social Welfare (MHSW) in Monrovia. A total of twenty-five copies of Instrument 02 were administered on public and private sector health institutions, of which nineteen were found usable, representing a response rate of 76%. Fifteen copies of Instrument 03 were administered on national and international NGOs operating in the country, of which nine were returned and seven found usable thereby representing a response rate of 47%. Among the documents consulted for data collection in Liberia were the National Health Policy (NPH), Report on the Drafts of New Law Provisions for the Health System, and the Draft Bill in Support of the National Health System.

9.2 The Role of Government

The MHSW is the only government agency responsible for health care under conflict in Liberia. However, intra-sectoral collaboration of health care issues at the national level is promoted through an *ad hoc* committee, the Technical Advisory Committee (TAC) and the Health Services Coordinating Committee (HSCC). The TAC includes senior representatives of the MHSW, the WHO, UNICEF and other development partners. Representation on the HSCC includes all members of the fourteen County Health Teams (CHTs) and NGOs participating in the health sector (MHSW, 2000). At the county operational level, the CHTs conduct meetings that are aimed at improving health services provision, developing joint plans of action, and agreeing on solutions to problematic programme areas. Our survey revealed that the relationship between the MHSW and members of the HSCC has been cordial and that NGOs are perceived as contributing immensely to national development. However, the coordinating activities of the Ministry does not appear to be effective enough as it will be seen later in this chapter that one of the recommendations of our survey is that the coordinating activities of the Ministry should be strengthened.

MHSW (2000) asserts that the effects of the Liberian civil war (1989-1997) had far-reaching effects that would be felt for generations. Apart from estimated deaths of between 150,000-200,000 out of a population of 2.6 million, other consequences of the conflict included:

- massive displacement of the population;
- destruction of productive capacity and physical infrastructures;
- aggravation of social problems;
- acceleration of the spread of communicable diseases;
- significant militarization of the population and the introduction of a 'culture' of violence;
- fractionalization and polarization of the countryside;
- considerable weakening of the central government authority;
- problems associated with demobilization and the slow transition process to a democratic government; and
- weakening of economic management capacity and breakdown in the provision of social services.

These impacts placed a lot of stress on the health sector. Thus, health facilities became poorly equipped, dilapidated, maldistributed and acutely in short supply. Besides, the quality of the available health services was limited and compromised by effects of destruction and vandalism. These led significantly to the underutilization of government services. Access to health services was also constrained by limited public transport and poor road network.

One of the effects of the conflict in Liberia is the significant increase in the number of orphanages for meeting the needs of children who lost their parents in the war or were neglected and/or abandoned. MHSW (2000) also asserted that the civil war led to the worsening maldistribution of health facilities and resources, characterized by gross inequalities in both urban and rural areas. It also aggravated the curative bias of the health system despite the overwhelming need for preventive, promotive and rehabilitative services and programmes. This is in agreement with the views expressed by the literature of post-conflict health, which states that one of the effects of the conflict on the health

80

system is the diversion of resources to the provision of acute curative care for war-related health conditions (Macrae, Zwi and Forsythe, 1995a).

The role of the Government of Liberia (GOL) to meaningfully intervene in solving these ensuing problems is constrained by the non-availability of funds. For example, MHSW (2000) observed that the post-war health budgets of the GOL were much lower than the pre-war budgets. Public allocation to health in 1981 was 10.2% of the total budget. However, in 1990, during the war, it was 5.6% of a smaller national budget. During the war, the document asserted, the only veritable spending on health by the public sector was on payment of salaries. However, since 1997, the GOL had been appropriating 15% of its budget to health, but the disbursements have been slow and much lower than the approved budgets. Besides, the share of wages in disbursements has been very high with non-wage health expenditures generally below 10% of expenditures.

To meet the financing gap, the GOL had always sought refuge in emergency and humanitarian assistance provided by the country's growing and vibrant NGO sub-sector. For example, the spending of overseas development assistance in the health sector was characterized by MHSW (2000) as 'robust in comparison to public sector spending'. Thus, in 1998, donors financed the major share of spending in the health sector, estimated to be US$25.4 million. However, donor releases tended to be lower than allocations. In 1997, for example, when Liberia was allocated US$100.7million ODA, the disbursements were actually 23.7% lower than 1996, while disbursements since 1996 averaged 20% of pledges. Worse still, it is expected that such assistance would continue to fall, given changes in the country's assistance status and other considerations.

The GOL has developed an NHP, which envisages putting in place a health sector designed to:

- prioritize PHC services;
- transfer responsibility to lower health management levels;
- empower people to be more involved in their health care;
- nurture and strengthen partnerships for health development;
- mobilize local and external resources in support of health; and
- generate the political will to provide resources required for the effective implementation of health and social welfare programmes.

To achieve these laudable objectives, the GOL and its development partners were expected to spend US$4.79 per capita on health during the financial year (FY) 1999/2000, rising to US$6.01, US$7.54 and US$9.47 respectively during the FY2000/2001, FY2001/2002 and FY2002/2003.

After the war in 1998, the total number of health workers of the MHSW was 3,196, rising by 9.5% to 3,500 in 1999. Health professionals constituted 43.7%

of the staff of MHSW in 1998 dropping marginally to 42.9% in 1999. In 2000, the total staff strength of the Ministry grew by 12.2% over the 1999 figure to 3926 when health personnel constituted 46% of the total staff.

Immediately after the war in 1997, the budget of the MHSW was L$13.5 billion, rising to L$80.8 million in 1998 by nearly 500%. It increased to L$133.1 million in 1999 by about 6.5% more than the 1998 value, and peaked at L$180.0 million in 2000 (Table 9.1).

Table 9.1: Budget/Actual Expenditure of the MHSW, Liberia (Million, Liberian Dollars)

	1997	1998	1999	2000
Budget	13.5	80.8	133.1	181.0
Actual Expenditure	9.6	21.2	83.8	96.8
Actual/Budget (%)	71.1	26.2	˙ 63.0	53.5

Source: *Survey*

While actual expenditure grew during the period under study, it was usually less than the budgeted amount. In fact, while the former experienced growth throughout the period under review, the latter, grew only once (Fig.9.1). Thus between 1997 and 1998, when actual expenditure of MHSW grew by 120%, the proportion of budget that was actually spent fell from 71.1% to 26.2%, indicating a growth rate of – 44.9%. Similarly, when actual expenditure grew phenomenally by nearly 300% between 1998 and 1999, the proportion of the budget actually spent grew by 36.9% from 26.2% to 63.0%. Between 1999 and 2000 when the actual expenditure had a modest growth of 15.1%, the expenditure/budget ratio fell by 9.5% from 63.0% to 53.5%.

It is not surprising therefore that MHSW (2000) asserted that with the cessation of the civil crisis in Liberia, many activities of health facilities like drugs and medical supplies were met through emergency and humanitarian assistance which averaged US$2.1 million per annum during the period 1997-1999. In fact, the assistance was said to be the main source of financing the essential requirements of functioning health facilities as about 99% of funds earmarked for drugs and medical supplies were not disbursed nor were expended for the desired purpose.

This has demonstrated that the enormity of the problems confronting post-conflict health care in Liberia is of such gargantuan proportions that funds that are available to the GOL through budget provisions are grossly inadequate. The projected needs of the GOL to meet the targets for accomplishing the goals of the NHP, demonstrates this quite vividly.

Fig. 9.1: Growth of Expenditure and Expenditure/Budget Ratio

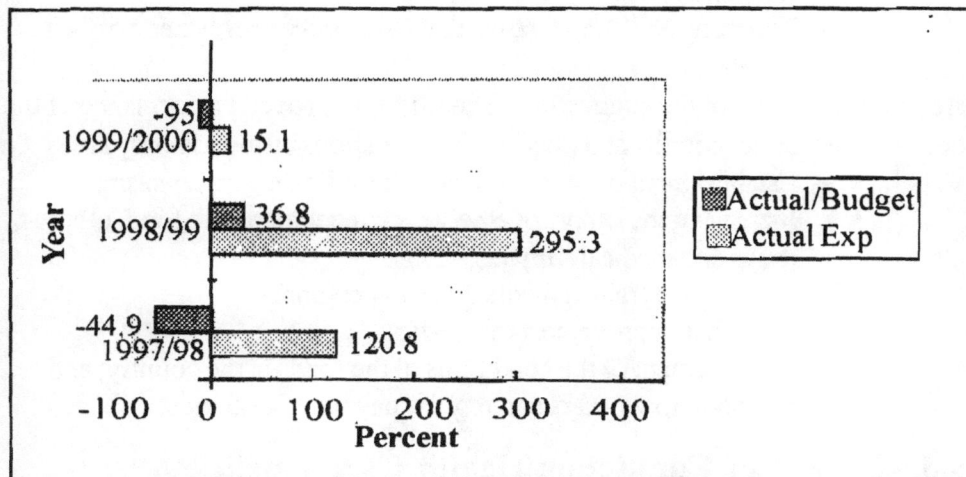

In this connection, the projected financing gap for the FY1999/2000 was estimated as US$23.43 million, dropping progressively to US$20.26 million in the FY2000/2001, US$16.27 million in FY 2001/2002 and US$11.27 million in FY2002/2003 (Table 9.2).

Table 9.2: Projected Financing Gap in Health Sector Finance Requirements for Meeting the Targets Set in the NHP of Liberia (US$ Million)

	FY 1999/2000	FY2000/2001	FY2001/2002	FY2002/2003
GDP	410.00	514.50	645.76	810.43
Total Budget	83.00	104.14	130.70	164.03
Health Sector Budget	12.45	15.62	19.61	24.61
Minimum Required	35.88	35.88	35.88	35.88
Financing Gap	23.43	20.26	16.27	11.27
US$ Per Capita Health Budget	4.97	6.01	5.74	9.47

Source: *MHSW (2000)*

Among the constraints identified by our survey as confronting the MHSW in successfully managing health care delivery under conflict and in post-conflict situations in Liberia are:

- Lack of logistics, especially vehicles;
- Poor road conditions especially during the rainy season;
- Overcrowded camp sites;

- · Inadequate emergency/relief items like food, drugs and medical supplies;
- Inadequate health personnel; and
- Too many NGOs and the resultant ineffective coordination of their activities.

Accordingly, some of the suggestions offered for improved performance of the health system under conflict and post-conflict situations by the Ministry are:

- Establishment of a more effective coordinating mechanism;
- Increasing the supply of emergency/relief items like food, utensils, drugs and medical supplies;
- Provision of trained medical/health personnel;
- Provision/improvement of logistics;
- Improvement of the conditions of the roads in the country; and
- Incentive to workers and regular payment of salaries.

9.3 Impact of Conflict on Health Care Facilities

We now analyze the effects of conflict on health care facilities in Liberia. We then compare our findings with prescriptions as it were from the literature of health care under conflict situations as well as those of other countries studied in this volume.

9.3.1 Characteristics of Respondent Facilities

The majority of the facilities that were surveyed (68.4%) were government-owned, while each of the for-profit, private sector and the not-for profit private sector/ NGOs owned 15.8% (Table 9.3). This contrasts sharply with the case of Sierra Leone (Chapter 10), where the majority of the health facilities that were surveyed belonged to the private sector. Most of the facilities that were surveyed operate at the secondary health care level, constituting 73.7% of the sample. Also, more facilities at the tertiary level (15.8%) were surveyed than at the primary level (10.5%). It is interesting that one of the tertiary institutions belonged to the not-for-profit private sector/NGOs. A Mission or such will likely own this. It is clear that as tertiary health care is capital intensive, the existence of a wealthy entrepreneurial class is a *sine qua non* to its establishment by the for-profit private sector. Given that Liberia, like Sierra Leone and Guinea-Bissau belong to the group of the forty-eight Least Developed Countries, according to the United Nations classification (see UN, 2002; for example); it is not unlikely that the 'tribe' of wealthy people will likely be many in the country and more particularly, in the health sector.

Table 9.3: Respondent Facilities by Type and Level of Care: Liberia

	Primary Health Care	Secondary Health Care	Tertiary Health Care	Total
Government/Public Sector	1(50.0)	10(71.4)	2(66.7)	13(68.4)
For-profit Private Sector	1(50.0)	2(14.3)	-	3(15.8)
Not-for profit Private Sector/NGOs/Missions	-	2(14.3)	1(33.3)	3(15.8)
Total	2(100.0) (10.5)	14(100.0) (73.7)	3(100.0) (15.8)	19(100.0) (100.0)

Source: *Survey*

Conflict began in most of the facilities surveyed (63.2%) in 1989 while for 36.8% of the facilities it started in 1990. For most of the facilities that were surveyed (89.5%), the conflict ended in 1997 while for a few (10.5%), it ended a year earlier (Table 9.4). A majority of these facilities (52.6%) experienced conflict for about eight years. However, unlike the case in Sierra Leone, none of the facilities that were surveyed reported that the conflict was on-going as at the time of the survey. The situation in Liberia at the time of our survey fits more into one of 'pure' post-conflict health care study.

Table 9.4: Distribution of Conflict Duration in the Facilities Surveyed in Liberia

Beginning/End	1996	1997	Total
1989	2(10.5)*	10(52.6)*	12(63.2)
1990	-	7(36.8)*	7(36.8)
Total	2(10.5)	17(89.5)	19(100.0)

*Percentage of Total
Source: *Survey*

9.3.2 *Effects on Human Resources, Other Resources and Service Operations*
(A) Human Resources

The effects of conflict on health personnel in the facilities that were surveyed in Liberia appear to be much for many personnel categories. For example, the average number of doctors per facility fell from 9.41 before the conflict to 8.00 during the first year of the conflict, a reduction of nearly 15% (Table 9.5). It dropped further by nearly 55% to 3.62 during the first year of the conflict. In the case of nurses, the effect appears even more drastic, the average number of nurses dropping from 38.5 per facility before the conflict by more than 76% to just 9.20 during the first year of the conflict, although it remained virtually at this value during the second year of the conflict. There appears to be a general shortfall in the number of pharmacists available in Liberia, if the data generated by this study, are anything to go by, since the average number of pharmacists per facility during the period under study tended to be about one! In spite of this, conflict still had the expected effect.

Table 9.5: Effects of Conflict on Staff (Average Number)*: Liberia

Variable	Before Conflict	Year 1 of Conflict	Year 2 of Conflict	Year 1 After Conflict	Year 2 After Conflict
Doctors	9.41	8.00	3.62	3.63	3.80
Nurses	38.53	9.20	9.10	9.11	20.1
Pharmacists	0.75	0.72.	0.71	0.68	1.42
Other Health Professional staff	71.53	45.14	42.22	44.56	54.80
Non-health Professional staff	86.44	14.53	14.10	14.15	15.40

* Rounding-off not done so as not to obscure the changes, even if marginal due to conflict.
Source: *Survey*

Thus the average number of pharmacists dropped from 0.75 per facility before the conflict to 0.72 during the first year of the conflict, a reduction of 4%. The supply of other health and non-health professionals was also adversely affected by the conflict. For example, the average number of other health professionals dropped from 71.53 before the conflict by nearly 38% to 45.14 during the first year of the conflict. Correspondingly, the average number of non-health professionals per facility dropped by over 83% from 86.44 before the conflict to 14.53 during the first year of the conflict!

The impact of peace on human resources in the facilities appears no less dramatic. The average number of doctors per facility increased marginally from 3.63 to 3.8 between the first and second years after the conflict, an increase of nearly 5%. Among nurses, the increase appears much more spectacular, not unlike the observed decrease due to the conflict. Thus, the average number of nurses per facility increased from 9.11 during the first year after the conflict by over 120% to 20.1 during the second year after the conflict. Even the average number of pharmacists increased from 0.68 to 1.42 between the first and second years after the conflict, an increase of 108%! There was also an improvement in the average number of other health professionals per facility after the cessation of hostilities from 44.56 to 54.80 during the same period, an improvement of about 23%. However, the increase in the average number of non-health professionals was less than the foregoing staff categories. On the whole, it can be concluded that the recent conflict in Liberia affected the supply of health personnel in the facilities adversely while cessation of hostilities had a salubrious effect on its supply.

(B)   Other Resources

The effects of conflict on the number of wards available for use in the facilities in Liberia cannot be said to be insignificant. For example, the average number of wards per facility studied decreased from 5.07 before the conflict to 4.54 during the first year of the conflict, a decrease of 10.5% (Table 9.6). However, between the first and second years of conflict, the effect appears marginal, the average number dropping 4.4% from 4.54 to 4.34. The effect on the average number of functioning wards appears more significant, dropping from 4.87 before the conflict to 3.77 during the first year of the conflict, a decrease of about 21.0%, which is about twice the decease in the proportion of wards available. Accordingly, the conflict in Liberia will be seen to have impaired health care services, with less availability of functioning wards.

On the other hand, the effect of peace was also salutary on the health infrastructure in Liberia. Our survey indicates that the available wards and the average number of functioning wards available per facility improved under post-conflict situations. For example, the average number of wards per facility increased by over 9% from 5.44 during the first year after the conflict to 5.94 during the second year after the conflict. The improvement in the average number of functioning wards was even more significant under a post-conflict situation than under conflict. It increased by over 24% from 4.36 during the first year after conflict to 5.42 during the second year after the conflict.

It is interesting that our survey, in two of the three years for which data were available, found out that the facilities that were surveyed spent more than the approved budget. This could mean two things: first that the facilities might be benefiting from unbudgeted assistance from donor agencies, or philanthropic and humanitarian organizations. This seems to corroborate the assertion of MHSW (2000) that ODA in the health sector of Liberia had been very robust in comparison to the public sector spending (p.23). The second possibility is that the data generated may be unreliable. Our conjecture is that the first reason appears more justifiable, particularly as the sample under study is dominated by secondary and tertiary facilities, which will likely have a better tradition of record keeping than primary facilities.

87

Table 9.6: Effects of Conflict on Other Resources and the Management Process (Average Number/Amount): Liberia

Variable	Before Conflict	Year 1 of Conflict	Year 2 of Conflict	Year 1 after Conflict	Year 2 after Conflict
Management meetings	9.20	9.40	6.70	6.71	8.68
Staff sent on training	0.38	0.36	0.30	0.32	1.73
Out-patients	34790	22330	21457	34569	45876
In-patients	1768	1354	1322	2549	2845
Wards	5.07	4.54	4.34	5.44	5.94
Functioning Wards	4.87	3.77	3.62	4.36	5.42
Budget (L$ Thousand)	70.65	152.65	145.62	-	-
Actual expenditure (L$ Thousands)	112.84	144.78	168.47	-	-
Expenditure/ Budget (%)	159.7	93.0	115.7	N/A	N/A

Source: *Survey*

Before the conflict, the average budget per facility was L$7.1 million, while the actual expenditure was L$11.3 million. This shows that on the average, each facility expended 60% more than its approved budget. This appears to be on the high side. However, it should be realized that second and tertiary facilities, which are capital-intensive in their operations, dominate the sample studied in Liberia. During the first year of conflict, the average budget rose by over 116% over the amount before the conflict. However, the expenditure/budget ratio declined to 93.0%. In the second year of conflict, the average budget per facility declined by nearly 5% to L$145,620 million. However, average expenditure rose by over 16% to L$168, 470 million per facility, giving an expenditure/ budget ratio of 115.7%. Our expectation that there should be a better stability in the data collection regime at the facility level was unmet by the lack of financial data at the facility level for the post-conflict years. This is very intriguing indeed.

(C) Management Processes and Service Operations

There was a marginal increase in the average number of management meetings held before the conflict and during the first year of the conflict: it increased from 9.20 to

9.40, an increase of 2.2%. However, when conflict set in, a significant reduction of the average number of management meetings held per facility was observed. Thus, the average number of management meetings held per facility fell from 9.40 during the first year of conflict by about 29% to 6.70 during the second year of the conflict. In Liberia, it appears that health facility staff tended to be not exposed to training. Thus, on average, in most cases, very much less than one health personnel attended training per year. In spite of this, the conflict still had its negative impact, however marginal. Thus, on average, there was a decrease of 5.3% (from 0.38 to 0.36) in the number of staff sent for training per facility before the conflict and during the first year of the conflict. Between the first and the second years of the conflict, the decrease in the proportion of staff who were not exposed to training widened by more than three times to 16.7%!

However, under post-conflict conditions, the situation improved. Thus the average number of staff who were sent for training per facility improved significantly by more than four times from 0.32 during the first year after the conflict to 1.73 during the second year after the conflict.

In Liberia, the conflict had negative effects on the attendance of health facilities by in-patients and outpatients. Before the beginning of the conflict, the average number of out-patients per facility was 34,790 per year. This fell to 22,330 during the first year of the conflict, a decrease of 35.8%. It fell further by 4% to 21,457 during the second year of the conflict. Similarly, the average number of in-patients per facility fell from 1,768 before the conflict by 23.4% to 1,354 during the first year of the conflict. It fell marginally further by 2.4% to 1,322 during the second year of the conflict. This seems to be at variance with the literature of health care delivery under conflict situations which expects that there will be a diversion of resources to treat more pressing war-related health problems proxied by increasing in-patient attendance during conflict. Our conjecture is that this may be due to inaccessibility problems created by the conflict for would-be patients.

On average, the health facilities that were surveyed were shut 1.71 times (about twice) during the conflict. Unfortunately, we did not collect data on how long the facilities were shut. Most facilities (42.1%) were shut twice while 21.2% were shut once. Facilities shut thrice were only 14.8% of the total while 5.3% of the facilities were shut four times (fig 9.2) This would have diminished the access of the population in the conflict areas to health care services during the conflict and would have contributed to the exacerbation of the morbidity and mortality of the people during this period.

Operators of health facilities perceived the conflict as having deleterious effects on health facilities and their operations. For example, in most facilities (94.7%), operators felt that the most adverse effects of the conflict on their operations were that, it leads to migration of staff. This is in agreement with our findings on the effects of conflict on the supply facility personnel in sub-section (A), above. The next most important adverse effect of conflict on the operations of health facilities is that it leads to an increase in the cost of production/operation (89.5%). Other effects are:

- Causing injuries to patients /staff (78.9%);
- Causing shut-down of operations (78.9%);
- Leading to increased deaths among patients/staff (73.7%);
- Causing destruction of equipment/facility (73.7%);
- Leading to increased disability of patient/staff (68.4%); and
- Causing general dislocation of facilities (63.2%).

To improve operations of the health care delivery system under conflict in Liberia operators of the respondent facilities offered the following suggestions:

- Enhance drug provision (73.7%);
- Improve working conditions of staff (73.7%);
- Provide health facilities in rural areas (57.9%);
- Governments and NGOs should increase funding of health care under conflict (47.4%); and
- Ensure that no organization has the monopoly of training (31.6%).

9.4 The Role of NGOs

Under conflict NGOs are known to play important roles in health care delivery. The extent to which this happened in Liberia constitutes what we analyzed in this sub-section. Only returns from seven of the fifteen NGOs surveyed in Liberia were found usable. All these NGOs happened to be international. Thus, no domestic NGO that was surveyed in Liberia returned usable administered survey instruments. Operations of these NGOs in the country appeared to be in response to the civil conflict that just ended in the country as only one (14.1%), was in operation in the country before 1990. We recall that the Liberian civil war started in 1989. Two each of the NGOs (28.6%) began operation in the country in 1991, 1996 and 1997.

The fact that most NGOs in Liberia were in operation in response to the demand of the ensuing conflict situations appears borne out by the data generated by our survey. Thus, no data were generated in relation to the operating staff before the conflict. The intensity of the conflict also appears to have an effect on the staff available for operation. In general, with greater conflict, the less is the average number of NGO staff in operation, suggesting that the intensity of hostilities inhibits freedom of NGO staff to operate. Thus, the average number of all categories of NGO personnel fell between the first year of the conflict and the second year of the conflict. The average health sector staff per NGO fell from 36 in the first year of the conflict by 6% to 34 during the second year of the conflict (Table 9.7). Some health sector staff appears more affected than others by the effect of conflict. The average number of doctors, for example, fell from 3.80 by nearly 16% during the first year of conflict to 3.20 during the second year of the conflict. The average number of nurses fell to about 7% from 17.40 to 16.30 between the first and second year of the conflict. In contrast, there was no change in the average number of pharmacists, which remained constant at 2.75 for both years.

The contributions of NGOs to health care delivery in Liberia will be better appreciated, if one considers the structure of health staff available in the health facilities vis-à-vis the NGOs. Of note is the fact that the average number of pharmacists in the facilities was much below the average number of pharmacists available per (international) NGO operating in the country. While on average there were 0.72 pharmacists per facility during the first year of the conflict, the corresponding value per NGO was 2.75, nearly four-fold. Similarly, on average, NGOs had more nurses than the health facilities operating in the country. The average number of nurses per NGO during the first year of the conflict in the country was, 17.40, which was nearly twice the average number (9.3) per facility. This further demonstrates that ODA was an important source of resource mobilization for health care delivery in Liberia, under the conflict.

. Peace also had a salubrious effect on the staffing pattern of NGOs operating in the health sector of Liberia. For example, the average total health staff per NGO increased from 35.21 in the first year after the conflict by about 21% to 42.43 in the second year after the conflict. Among the doctors, the corresponding increase was more spectacular, from 2.43 by 56% to 3.80. However, the increase in the average number of nurses is less dramatic: by nearly 11% from 10.71 to 11.85 during the same period. Next to doctors, the post-conflict situations in Liberia appear to favour the supply of pharmacists in NGOs more. The average number of NGO pharmacists increased by nearly 33% from 2.17 a year after the conflict to 2.88 during the second year after the conflict.

Our data show that the average amount spent per NGO in Liberia is somewhat much lower than average actual expenditure per facility. This confirms the earlier observation of MHSW (2000) as regards the robust contribution of ODA to health spending in Liberia. However, the average amount spent per NGO tended to decrease with increasing years of hostilities. This fell by about 3% to L$3.70 million during the second year of the conflict.

Table 9.7: NGO Health Personnel During and After Conflict: Liberia (Average Number)

Health Personnel	1st Year of Operation during Conflict	2nd Year Operation during Conflict	1st Year after Conflict	2nd Year after Conflict
Doctors	3.80	3.20	2.43	3.80
Nurses	17.40	16.20	10.71	11.85
Pharmacists	2.75	2.75	2.17	2.88
Other Health-Professional Staff	13.00	10.75	10.42	15.50
Non-health Professional Staff	21.00	18.60	18.65	23.57
Average Total Health Sector Staff	36.00	34.00	35.21	42.43

Source: *Survey*

This is in contrast to what happened in the health facilities where the average actual expenditure per facility actually rose by over 16% during the same period. This result appears rather intriguing. Since the facilities spent more than they budgeted, on average, it is felt that the surplus spent in the facilities must have come from donors, philanthropic organizations and NGOs. Yet, our results show that NGOs spent less on average than the facilities. However, there may not be a contradiction in the findings, as the amount under analysis actually referred to how much the NGOs spent *directly* on their health care delivery operations.

The NGOs that were surveyed in Liberia believe that a conflict has negative effects that are inimical to the operations of the health sector. Among these are:

- Non-availability of drugs/expired drugs/high cost of drugs (100%);
- Increased health hazards/recurrence of epidemics (100%);
- Loss of staff resulting from staff migration, death or layoff (57.1%); and
- Destruction of health facilities/equipment (57.1%).

The NGOs were also asked to identify problems and constraints experienced in the delivery of health care while under conflict. These include:

- Lack of equipment/clinics/reconstruction of damaged facilities (85.7%);
- Lack of qualified staff (85.7%);

- Lack of security (85.7%);
- Poor logistics (85.7%); and
- High cost/short supply of drugs (71.4%).

Among the suggestions offered by the NGOs for improving health delivery under conflict situations in Liberia were:

- Ensuring the supply of cheaper drugs (100%);
- Community mobilization/restoration of local authorities (85.7%);
- Increased donor assistance (85.7%);
- Equipping more hospitals/clinics (71.4%); and
- Improving logistics (71.4%).

It is not clear, how effective the HSCC of the MHSW is, in coordinating the activities of NGOs, particularly NNGOs involved in health delivery under conflict and in post-conflict situations in the country, in order to reduce waste, duplication and redundancies. In particular, the problems of sanctions imposed on the government of President Taylor for his alleged involvement in fueling the Sierra Leonean civil war, suggests many NNGOs would rather deal more with domestic NGOs than the government in their attempt to assist the country overcome the problems of post-conflict health care. The shortage of qualified personnel in the MHSW, suggests the country would not have the capacity to coordinate and monitor the activities of NGOs involved in health care delivery under conflict and in post-conflict situations in the country. Accordingly, it will be difficult, under present circumstances, for Liberia to contain the Macrae (1997) critical rehabilitation dilemmas confronting post-conflict health care.

9.5 Health System Performance

Overall, the poor ranking given to it by many international publications captures the impact of conflict on the health system of Liberia. For example, the *World Health Report, 2000*, published by WHO, ranked the overall health system of the country 186th among 191 nations, that is sixth from the bottom. Using the other eight performance measures, the publication ranked Liberia on various measures as follows:

- Health level (proxied by Disability-adjusted Life Expectancy- DALE): 181st;
- Health distribution: 191st;
- System responsiveness level: 175th – 176th;
- System responsiveness distribution: 176th;
- Fairness in financial distribution: 84th – 86th;
- Overall goal attainment: 187th;
- Health expenditure per capita: 181st; and
- Performance on health level: 176th.

Besides, Liberia, like Guinea-Bissau and Sierra Leone are classified as belonging to a group of countries of Africa and Asia where the population transition has not taken place.

For example, the total fertility of the country between 1995-2000 was 6.80, up from 6.29 for 1959-1965 (UN, 2002). This continues to put pressure on the country's inadequate health infrastructure, worsened by years of conflict. In all, a lot still needs to be done to see that the health system of Liberia measures up to standard. Given the fact that the government is hard-pressed, particularly during conflict, in living up to its obligation in the health sector, the country will still need the assistance of the domestic and external private sector, bilateral and multilateral organizations in raising the required resources to rehabilitate and develop the country's war-ravaged health system.

9.6 Summary, Implications and Recommendations

The civil war in Liberia appears to be the longest so far. In spite of the holding of elections, the government of President Charles Taylor has been under serious attack by another batch of rebels. In fact, at the time of putting finishing touches to the writing of the study report, President Taylor, according to his agreement with the rebels, had stepped down, and his deputy sworn-in as the President pending the formation of an interim government made up of technocrats who will organize democratic elections. Nigeria offered President Taylor political asylum to facilitate the roadmap to peace in Liberia. However, sporadic fighting still existed in the hinterland of the country, in spite of this development.

The MHSW is the only government agency responsible for health care under conflict and in post-conflict situations in Liberia, but intra-sectoral collaboration of health care issues at the national level is promoted through an *ad hoc* committee, the Technical Advisory Committee (TAC) and the Health Services Coordinating Committee (HSCC). The TAC includes senior representatives of the MHSW, the WHO, UNICEF and other development partners. Representation on the HSCC includes all members of the fourteen County Health Teams (CHTs) and NGOs participating in the health sector (MHSW, 2000). At the county operational level, the CHTs conduct meetings aimed at improving health services provision, developing joint plans of action, and agreeing on solutions to problematic programme areas. While our survey revealed that the relationship between the MHSW and members of the HSCC has been cordial, it is very doubtful if the HSCC, as constituted, is capable of coordinating the activities of NGOs effectively with a view to avoiding duplication of activities, wastages and redundancies and hence make their interventions sustainable.

The GOL is constrained severely in meeting the challenges of post-conflict health care delivery shortage of funds. Thus, its post-war health budgets were much lower than the pre-war budgets. Public allocation to health in 1981, for example, was 10.2% of the total budget. However, in 1990, during the war, it was 5.6% of a smaller national budget. During the war, the only veritable spending on health by the public sector was on payment of salaries. To bridge the financing gap, the GOL depends on foreign assistance of different forms.

In most of the facilities surveyed (63.2%), the conflict began in 1989 while for 36.8% of the facilities, the conflict started in 1990. For most of the facilities (52.6%), the conflict lasted for eight years. For the remaining facilities the conflict lasted for seven years. Many of the facilities that were surveyed reported being exposed to varying degrees of closure resulting from the conflict. On average, facilities were shut 1.71 times. Most facilities (42.1%) were shut twice during the conflict while 21.2 % were shut once. Only 14.8% of the facilities were shut three times and the proportion of facilities shut four times during the conflict was just 5.3%.

The conflict had varying effects on the supply of the different facility personnel categories. For example, the average number of doctors fell by nearly 15% during the first year of the conflict dropping further by 55% during the second year of the conflict. However, with nurses, the effect is more drastic, with the average number of nurses dropping from 38.5 per facility before the conflict by more than 76% to just 9.20 during the first year of the conflict, although it remained virtually at this value during the second year of the conflict. The impact of peace is heart-warming as the supply of health personnel at the facilities, particularly for nurses, where the average number per facility increased by over 120% between the first year after the conflict and the second year after the conflict.

The average number of functioning wards decreased by 21% during the first year of conflict. With the cessation of conflict the situation improved. The average number of functioning wards, increased by 24% from 4.36 between the first year after the conflict to 5.42 during the second year after the conflict. The conflict has also taken its toll on the management process in the health facilities. The number of management meetings held per facility decreased by 29% from 9.40 during the first year of conflict to 6.70 during the second year after the conflict. A decrease was also observed in the average number of staff exposed to training as a result of the conflict. For example, the average number of staff exposed to training fell by 16.7% between the first year of the conflict and the second year of the conflict. With the cessation of hostilities, the situation improved. Thus, the average number of staff sent for training was more than 440% between the first year after the conflict and the second year after the conflict.

Most of the NGOs that were studied began operations in the country in response to the problems posed by the conflict, as only 14.1% of them were in operation before the conflict began. NGOs boosted health care delivery under the conflict and in post-conflict situations particularly, by enhancing the supply of health personnel where the country suffered critical shortages. While the average number of pharmacists per facility was between 0.71 and 0.75 particularly just before and during the conflict, the corresponding average number of pharmacists per NNGO studied was 2.71 and 2.75 a multiple of nearly three times. Similarly, the average number of nurses per NGO was about twice that per facility. However, our data suggest that the average amount spent per NGO was lower than what was spent per facility.

A major implication of our study is that Liberia appears to be worse off in terms of funds availability when compared with other conflict countries. This is particularly the case when it is compared with others it appears to have received less from NGOs. In fact, government documents confirm that in general, even at the bilateral and multilateral level, donor releases tended to be less than what was promised. Liberia requires a lot of support and it deserves such support, not only for post-conflict health care, but also for the establishment of enduring peace. Of the three conflict countries studied, it is particularly more vulnerable to relapse into violence.

Liberia's institutional and legal framework for health care delivery both under conflict and in post-conflict situations does not appear to be well developed. There is a need to develop these and more importantly, there is a need to have a mechanism for coordinating the activities of foreign agencies who are assisting in funding health care delivery under conflict and in post-conflict situations with a view to minimizing the duplication of efforts, wastages and redundancies and ensuring sustainability of the interventions.

Our study reveals that the country lacks adequate human capital for post-conflict health care delivery. This is complicated, as it does not have the appropriate institutions and agencies for building human capital for providing health care delivery under conflict and in post-conflict situations. Efforts should be made to build the necessary human capacity through short-term and professional training, using in particular, institutions that are available within the sub-region. Where this cannot be obtained, training from outside the subregion can then be sought.

---

[1] At the time of finishing the report, the Liberian civil war II was in progress. The rebels have succeeded in unseating the elected government of President Charles Taylor. He sought political asylum in Nigeria and a new government led by his former Vice President was sworn into office. A fresh attempt to have an international peace-keeping force involving the United Nations and ECOWAS had been put in place.

Chapter Ten

ASSESSING POST-CONFLICT HEALTH CARE IN SIERRA LEONE

10.1 Introduction

The fieldwork for Sierra Leone was done during the last quarter of 2001. A stratified random sample procedure was used to select facilities to reflect the relative distribution between public and private facilities; the different levels of operation that is primary, secondary and tertiary health care; and the areas operation, whether urban or rural. A total of fifty-nine of the three types of structured questionnaires were distributed, made up of one of Instrument 01; as only one government agency, the Ministry of Health and Sanitation is involved in health care delivery under conflict or in situations of emergency; thirty-six of Instrument 02 out of which twenty-seven with usable responses were returned. This represented a response rate of 75%. As for Instrument 03, a total of twenty questionnaires were distributed with thirteen usable questionnaires returned. This represents a response rate of 65%. The study team met many stakeholders in the health sector of the country. They included the Director-General of Medical Services who is the professional head of the Health Department in the Ministry of Health and Sanitation; the Secretary of Medical Research Ethics; the Head, Policy Management and Implementation Unit of the Ministry; the Public Relations Officer of the Ministry; and the Head, NGO Coordination Unit.

One of the major problems encountered by the study team was the general display of reluctance by respondents to take part in the study. Consequently, enumerators had to make several visits to obtain useful responses. In particular, respondents were particularly reluctant to provide financial information, despite the assurance of confidentiality.

10.2 The Role of Government

The Ministry of Health and Sanitation is the only government agency involved in health care delivery under conflict or emergency situations. However, there is a unit of the Ministry, which coordinates the activities of NGOs. Among such NGOs are the Sierra Leone Red Cross Society, Save the Children of Sierra Leone, Caritas Makeni, Care International; Leones and Cents and Planned Parenthood Association of Sierra Leone.

Even before the beginning of hostilities, the health care delivery system of Sierra Leone had reached an appalling state of deterioration in quality and scope. Not a single Government Hospital was functioning effectively. For example, Connaught Hospital, the biggest referral hospital in the country presented the sight of a severely overused institution with structures and facilities completely decayed or in a severe state of disrepair. Several toilet and running water systems did not function; beds and mattresses were in a deplorable state, and there were no beddings; the operating threatres rarely functioned; and sterilization facilities were almost zero; the laundry facilities were out of operation for more than six years; laboratory facilities also were non- functional while the X-ray unit needed urgent upgrading and adequate staffing. Besides, the Eye Clinic also required complete rehabilitation and the dental unit was rather out of date and needed a more congenial surrounding (ROS, 1993).

Under, the situation described above, the role of the Government of the Republic of Sierra Leone (GOROS), was to lead the way in the rehabilitation of the wards of the different hospitals, supported by individuals and business houses within the country. Funds were also obtained from Development Finance Institutions like the African Development Bank (ADB) and the World Bank. Indeed, ROS (1993) reported that the ADB earmarked some funds for the rehabilitation of nine hospitals throughout the country and that the World Bank would provide support for the upgrading of hospitals in various parts of the country through its Health and Population Project. In terms of improvement in drug supplies, the World Health Organization (WHO) and the United Nations Children's Fund (UNICEF) supported funding the cost recovery programme of government. In particular, as a participant in the Bamako Initiative in which African Ministers of Health committed their countries to health finance reforms and promotion of community participation in the management of health care delivery, the GOROS, is expected to promote decentralization of decision-making, dialogue and improved participation of the different stakeholders of health care delivery both in peace time and under conflict. Unfortunately however, the country tends to spend less than 1% of its total budget on the health sector. In fact, ROS (1993) asserted that Sierra Leone is the only country in the world with such disproportionate health expenditure. Indicative of such low spending is the fact that in 1993, less than six ambulances were road-worthy in the country! However, WHO National Health Accounts (NHA) Data Files (2000) estimated the total health expenditure of Sierra Leone in 1997 to be 4.9% of the GDP. Government expenditure on health as a proportion of total health expenditure was estimated at 9.7%. This contrasts poorly with that of other countries under conflict in Africa like Liberia (66.7%), Guinea-Bissau (75.6%), Mozambique (71.3%) and Rwanda (50.1%). This suggests that the burden of health care financing is on other sources of health funds like households, firms and donor agencies.

GOROS has responsibility for the development and implementation of the National Health Policy (NHP). The first was developed in 1993 and it has specific goals for different areas of health care delivery and management like administration; financing; manpower development; infrastructure and transportation; primary health care; secondary and tertiary health care; private practice; drugs and medical supplies; control of communicable diseases; nutrition; information system and education; and legal aspects of health, among others. In terms of administration, for example, the goal of the NHP is to decentralize the administrative structure of the health care delivery system culminating in the creation of district, provincial, and area health boards, which will only function within the framework of less stringent central control. Similarly, in the area of financing, it seeks to identify areas of possible mobilization of resources to ensure sustainability.

The National Health Action Plan (NHAP), which was developed in 1994 (ROS, 1994), builds on the NHP and it outlines the main steps needed to develop a more effective, efficient and equitable health system. It gave decentralization of the health system top priority. This will involve the creation of new leadership teams at lower levels, like the district level to be headed by district medical officers (public health) or district medical officers (clinical). At this level, the NHAP seeks to give additional training in the skills of the Community Health Officers to staff at the district level without primary health skills. As part of the decentralization process, the NHAP proposed the provision of a basic range of facilities at the village level and a wider range at health centres located in chiefdom headquarters and small towns. This document also seeks to promote cooperation and dialogue between government and NGOs with a view to translating the latter's useful and welcome support in a more positive and operationally more transparent perspective. The total cost of the NHAP was estimated as nearly $300 million over a five-year period. About half of the estimated cost is represented by capital expenditure. Of the total cost, 13% was estimated to come from GOROS while 24% was expected from donor agencies, leaving a huge financing gap of 63%. The expectation of nearly twice the contribution of government from donor agencies to finance the NHAP is in agreement with our earlier finding that the burden of health financing in Sierra Leone is more on other sources of health care funds than government.

Under conflict, our study shows that the situation was compounded. Human, physical and technical resources were expectedly, one of the first victims of conflict. For example, ROS (1993) showed that even before conflict, the number of health personnel in the country was very limited. There were a total of 203 medical officers or one per 17,000 population, 58 public health specialists or one per 61,000 population. It is worse in some specialist areas. There was only a total of five peadiatricians or one per 703, 000 population while there were only twenty-seven surgeons or one per 130,000 population. While we did not have access to aggregate data on the situation under conflict, our survey of facilities suggests that conflict affected health personnel adversely, resulting in staff migration, loss of staff through death and/or layoff of staff. Additionally, health facilities and equipment were also destroyed, therefore the immediate impact of the inability of the country to meet the set targets of government in the NHAP failed woefully. For example, it would be impossible to meet the strategic manpower targets set out in this document where, it was proposed to have at least one health staff per facility in all the PHC staff categories like Community Health Officers and Nurse/Midwife, for example. The Action Plan calls for meeting the gap of a total of 1,060 PHC staff of different categories over a five-year period. Another impact of conflict in the health manpower system of Sierra Leone is the inability of government to operate the priorities of manpower development, particularly in relation to the effective distribution and utilization of all categories of health personnel. The impact of conflict on the manpower system, therefore, in depleting the meager resources available will make meeting these targets a mirage, thereby making the required role of government in this regard more of an up-hill task.

Our survey also reveals that the breakdown of law and order as a result of the conflict led to the inability to operate the management framework proposed by the NHP and NHAP as part of the policy reforms of the health sector in the country. Part of the effects is the inability of communities to participate actively in the operation of the Bamako Initiative, particularly as regards seeking alternative means of financing drug provision in health facilities at the PHC level as well as the operation of user-charges and exemption schemes. Government monitoring functions in the health care sector particularly those relating to disease surveillance, disease prevention and control are also adversely affected by conflict (Macreae, Zwi and Forsythe, 1995b). Besides, we found that closure of facilities is, perhaps, the most important impact of conflict in health care delivery in the country. Accordingly, there would be a fewer facilities to coordinate and monitor, if any. Where there were facilities operating, emphasis would be shifted to curative care to the detriment of other aspects of health care like preventive care and public health, in general. Government was therefore unable to fulfill its expected role. As there is no specific agency of government charged with post-conflict health care *ab initio*, it is difficult to see how government could 'short circuit' the ensuing problems.

10.3 Impact of Conflict on Health Care Facilities

The literature of health delivery under conflict states that health facilities constitute a major part of the health system that suffers adverse consequences as a result of conflict. Among such consequences are the destruction and/or neglect of health facilities; looting of the facilities and diversion of resources to the provision of acu.e are for war-related health problems (Zwi and Ugade, 1989; and Macrae, Zwi and Forsythe, 1995b). The extent of the impact of conflict in the health facilities of Sierra Leone is analyzed in the next sub-section.

10.3.1 *Characteristics of Respondent Facilities*
The majority of the facilities that were surveyed and whose questionnaires were usable (16 or 59.2%) belonged to the private sector. In particular, twelve or 44.4% were operated in the for-profit private sector while the balance of four or 14.8% belonged to the NGOs/Missions or the not-for-profit private sector. Only eleven or 40.7% were government-owned (Table 10.1). In terms of level of health care delivery, most (77.7%) were at the PHC level 11.1% of them were each at secondary or tertiary levels. Expectedly, all tertiary level facilities in the sample are government-owned, given the high capital-intensity of such level, which may not make it attractive for private-sector investment.

Table 10.1: Respondents Facilities by Type and Level of Care: Sierra Leone

Ownership/Level	Primary	Secondary	Tertiary	Total
Government	7(33.3)*	1(33.3)	3(100.0)	11(40.7)
Private Sector (For Profit)	11(52.4)	1(33.3)	-	12(44.4)
NGOs/Missions (Not-for-Profit Private Sector)	3(14.3)	1(33.3)	-	4(14.8)
Total	21(100.0) (77.7)	3(99.9)** (11.1)	3(100.0) (11.1)	27(99.9)** (100.0)

Note: * *Numbers in parenthesis are percentages.*
   ** *Round-off error.*
Source: *Survey*

The conflict began in most of the facilities providing relevant information, in 1991. Only thirteen of the twenty-seven facilities with usable questionnaires provided information on this part of the study. It was only in one case that it began in 1992. The conflict was rather prolonged in that only in one case did it last for eight years. For the majority (69.2%), it lasted for nine years. In one case, the conflict lasted for ten years while it was still on-going at the time of the survey in one other case. In fact, in the case of the single facility where conflict began in 1992, it lasted till the year 2000, a total of eight years (Table 10.2). It is interesting that this result suggests that respondents viewed the military regime of Captain Valentine E. M. Strasser as being within the period of conflict.

Table 10.2: Distribution of the Beginning and End of Conflict in the Facilities Surveyed

Beginning/End	1999	2000	2001	On-going	Total
1991	1(7.7)*	9(69.2)	1(7.7)	1(7.7)	12(92.3)
1992	-	1(7.7)	-	-	-
Total	1(7.7)	10(76.9)	1(7.7)	1(7.7)	13(100.0)

Source: *Survey*

10.3.2 *Effects of Conflicts on Human and Other Resources, Management Processes and Service Operations*

(A) Human Resources

The literature of health care under conflict, suggests that human resources are one of the first victims of the effects of conflict on health facilities. Such effects are: (e)migration of skilled personnel; death, repression or assault of health staff; and general feeling of insecurity, which may prevent staff from performing their legitimate functions. The effect of conflicts on staff in the facilities that were surveyed appears to depend on the category of staff. There does not appear to be a drastic reduction in the average number of staff per facility between the start of conflict and just before it. However, in general, there appears to be some reduction, however slight. There was, on average, a reduction from the number of doctors from 3.6 a year before the conflict to 2.6 during the first year of the conflict. Other non-health professionals also experienced a similar trend in decline (Table 10.3). In the case of a country with a long period of conflict like Sierra Leone, the expected decline may come later in the conflict. This is one of the limitations of the study, which uses the same instrument to collect data from countries with varying experiences in conflict including the period for which the conflict lasted. In the case of nurses and pharmacists, the change does not appear to be glaring. Between the first year of the conflict and the beginning of the conflict cessation, some changes in the average number of health staff that were available per facility were also observable. Thus, among doctors, a slight decline from 2.6 to 2.4 can be observed. Among nurses, there was an observed average reduction from 9.5 to 9.3. However, following closely with what the literature expects is the reduction among 'other health professionals' and 'non-health professionals'.

In the case of the former, there was a reduction from an average of four in the first year of the conflict to 2.4 at the beginning of cessation of the conflict, a reduction of 40%. In the case of the latter, the corresponding reduction was from an average of 5.7 to 4.2 (a reduction of 16%).

What is more interesting is that, during the first year after the conflict and the second year after the conflict, the change in the average number of staff available in the facilities, was more glaring. For example, the average number of doctors increased from 2.4 to 3.7 or 54%. Among nurses, the change is dramatic, increasing from an average of 9.3 by over 124% to 20.9. Similarly, more dramatic observations can be made about the increase in the number of pharmacists, other health professionals and other non-health professionals after the cessation of the conflict. In the case of pharmacists, the average number during the first year after the conflict increased from three to seven by over 208%; other health professionals increased from an average of 2.4 to 4.4 (by over 183%) while non-health professionals increased from an average of 4.2 by about 260% to 15.1. Thus, peace engendered the supply of health professionals as expected in Sierra Leone.

Table 10.3: Effects of Conflict on Staff (Average Number)*

Staff Type	Before Conflict	Year1 of Conflict	Year 1 After Conflict	Year 2 After Conflict
Doctors	3.6	2.6	2.4	3.7
Nurses	9.7	9.5	9.3	20.9
Pharmacists	1.8	2.1	3.0	7.0
Other Health Professionals	4.8	4.0	2.4	4.4
Non-Health Professionals	6.0	5.7	4.2	15.1

*Rounding-up not done so as not to mask the changes observed.
Source: *Survey*

(B) Other Resources
There was a limited change in the average number of wards available in facilities as a result of the conflict. Thus, the average number of wards decreased from 6.4 before the conflict to 6.1 during the first year of conflict, a decrease of about 5.0%. The effect of the conflict appears slightly more on the availability of functioning wards. This decreased from an average of 6.2 before the conflict to 5.8 during the first year of the conflict, representing a decrease of about 7% (Table 10.4). The cessation of hostilities also had some salutary effects on the number of wards

available per facility as well as the number of functioning wards. This resulted in increase in the average number of wards available from six at the inception of the cessation of the conflict to 6.9 during the second year after the conflict, an increase of 15%. Also, the corresponding average number of functioning wards improved by over 12% from 5.7 to 6.4. As noted earlier, there was a general reluctance among respondents to provide financial information. The study sought information from facilities as regards their approved budget and their actual expenditure. In addition, it sought information about their source of raising funds through government budget, revenue generated, philanthropy/ NGOs (domestic and foreign), and other sources. However, only one facility 'volunteered' information as it were, and for most times, it was the same figure of 3.0 million Leones of the budget and actual expenditure and this is regarded as unreliable.

However, in terms of information on the total funds collected from various sources, between six and eight of the facilities provided information. However, the information was not disaggregated. For example, eight facilities provided information on their total funds before the conflict, with a minimum of 1.0 million Leones, maximum of 3.9 million Leones, a mean of 2.45 million Leones and a standard deviation of 1.2 million Leones. During the first year of the conflict, the number of facilities supplying information dropped to six with a ridiculously low minimum value of 10,000 Leones, a maximum of 6.0 million Leones and a mean of 2.74 million Leones. Six facilities supplying information on their total funding from all sources with a mean funding of 1:58 million Leones, a minimum of 1,000 million Leones and a maximum of 3.25 million Leones. However, it is intriguing to note that there was no facility-supplied information on the total funding for the first or second year after the conflict.

Notwithstanding, the resulting limitation of the data, and the information supplied, appears to paint a familiar picture of the effects of violence on the record-keeping, information-gathering, analysis, storage and retrieval as well as the funding of health care facilities. As expected, there is a fall in the mean total funding with the advent of conflict. Also, the conflict is expected to affect the information gathering and record-keeping system of the facilities, caused particularly for the shutting down of operations. This may in fact, account, in part, for the inabilities of the facilities to provide the required information apart from the usual reluctance of respondents to provide financial information in surveys. As will be seen later, in this chapter, two out of three of the facilities that were surveyed were shut down, at least twice during the conflict while about 89% of them were shut down, at least once.

Table 10.4: Effects of Conflict on Management Process and Other Resources* (Average Number)

Variables	Before Conflict	Year 1 of Conflict	Year 1 after Conflict	Year 2 after Conflict
Management Meetings	6.6	4.7	3.7	8.6
Staff sent on Training	3.0	2.6	2.4	1.7
Out-patients	1170	1438.6	1347.9	1107.2
In-patients	205.8	1106.8	919.3	661.7
Wards	6.4	6.1	6.0	5.9
Functioning Wards	6.2	5.8	5.7	6.4

*Rounding-off not done so as not to mask the effect of change.
Source: *Survey*

(C) Management Processes and Service Operations

The management process of the health system and of facilities as well as uninterrupted operations of health care delivery at facility levels are major victims of conflict. Interruption in the management process at the facility level can be measured by the frequency of management meetings, and the number of members of staff exposed to training and capacity building opportunities. As expected, there is a decline in the frequency of management meetings with conflict in the facilities surveyed in Sierra Leone. Thus, the average number of management meetings held decreased from 6.6 before the conflict by about 29% to 4.7 in the first year of the conflict. Also, on the average, fewer staff were exposed to training and capacity development with the conflict. Before the conflict, on average, three staff per facility attended training in the year. This dropped to 2.6, a decrease of over 13%, in the first year of the conflict. With the cessation of hostilities, there was a marked improvement in the average number of management meetings per facility. Thus, the average number of management meetings increased by over 132% from 3.7 one year after the conflict to 8.6, two years after the conflict. However, the expected improvement, in the number of staff exposed to training and capacity development did not materialize. Rather than an increase, a fall is observed; it fell by 29% from an average of 2.4 per facility, a year after the conflict to 1.7, two years after the conflict. This is in spite of the fact that more staff were in position, two years after the conflict. This may need investigation, but possible causes may include lack of funds or non-availability of the type of training needed for the resulting overwhelming number of staff. This may also be due to the lingering effects of the activities of the RUF with respect to the indiscriminate amputation of limbs and hands during the war, thus instilling fear into the populace.

A proxy for determining the effects of conflict on services delivery at the facility level is determining its effects on the number of in-patients, and out-patients treated at the facility and the number of times the facilities were shut down. The literature suggests an increase in both out-patients and in-patients for war-related health indications. In particular, Macrae, Zwi and Forsythe (1995b) suggest that conflict will result in the diversion of resources to the provision of acute care for war-related health problems. While there was a slight increase in the average number of out-patients from 1,170 before the conflict to 1438.6 (increase of 23%) in the first year of the conflict, there was an overwhelming increase of over 437% in the average number of in-patients from 205.8 before the conflict to 1106.8 during the first year of the conflict. This agrees with what the literature says about the diversion or resources to acute care of war-related health conditions. With the cessation of hostilities, there was a fall in the average number of both out-patients and in-patients, as expected. Thus, the average number of out-patients fell from 1347.9 during the first year after the conflict by nearly 18% to an average of 1107.2, two years after the conflict. The average number of in-patients also fell by 28% from 919.3, a year after the conflict to 616.7, two years after the conflict.

On average, the facilities surveyed were shut 1.78 times (or about twice) during the conflict. In particular, 22.2% of them were shut down once, 48.1%, twice 14.8% three times and 3.7% four times (Fig. 10.1). This would have adverse effects on the health of the people and could have led to increased mortality during the conflict.

We also surveyed the perceptions of the facility operators as to what were the effects of conflicts on the operations of the various facilities. The most serious effect as perceived by our respondents is that conflict leads to closures of facilities (92.6%). Next in the order of importance is that it results in increased disability of patients/staff, while migration of staff, destruction of equipment, increased cost of operation all share the third position with 74.1% of respondents indicating such views. Other effects are: increased death among patients/ staff (59.3%); injury to patients and staff (44.4%); and general dislocation of facilities (29.6%).

Fig. 10.1: Conflict and Closure of Facilities

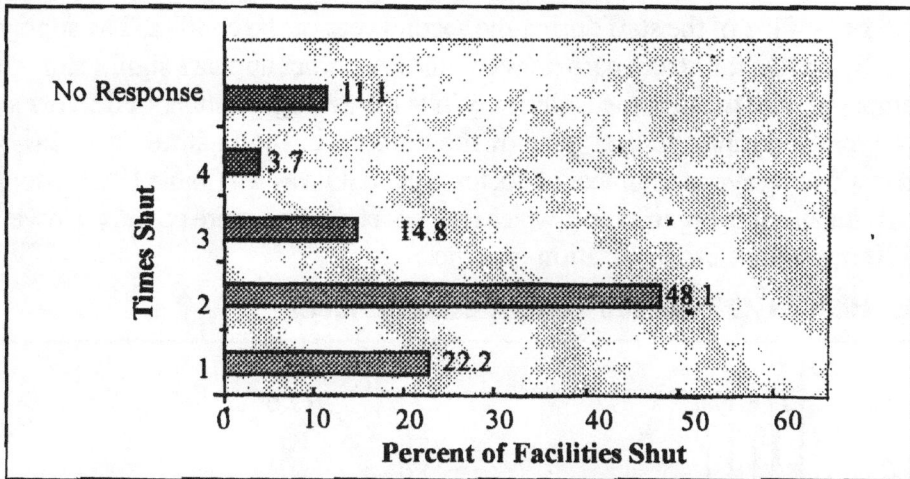

As a way of improving the management and operations of health facilities under conflict, the respondents offered the following suggestions:

- Improve working conditions of staff (70.4%);
- Enhance drug provision (66.7%);
- Provide rural health facilities (33.3%);
- Government and NGOs should increase funding (22.2%); and
- Ensure that nobody monopolizes training of staff (22.2%).

10.4   The Role of NGOs

NGOs play important roles in health in times of conflict in many countries of the world like Cambodia, Palestine, Afghanistan, Rwanda, Mozambique, Angola, to name a few. To what extent have they been of assistance in Sierra Leone? This is the essence of this part of the study. Of the twenty NGOs surveyed, seventeen usable questionnaires were retrieved, representing a response rate of 85%. Twelve (70.6%) of the NGOs were domestic while seven (or 41.2%) of them were founded after the commencement of the conflict in 1991. This suggests many of the NGOs were founded in response to the problems posed by conflict (Fig 10.2). In fact 50% of the domestic NGOs were founded after the commencement of hostilities. The corresponding portion of the foreign NGOs founded after the commencement of the conflict is just 20%.

The average number of staff used by the NGOs in the country depends on the period in relation to conflicts. Thus on average, total staff per organization was larger during the first year of conflict than during the second year. In the first year of the conflict, the average total staff of the NGOs operating in the country was 27.3[1]. This decreased to 24.9 or by 8.8% during the second year of the conflict.

107

During the first year after the conflict, an average total staff per NGO increased to 35.2 or by 41% of the staff during the second year of the conflict. The supply of staff by NGOs for health care delivery under conflict appears significant when compared with those in the facilities. While the average number of doctors staff per facility during the first year of the conflict in the facilities was 2.6, the corresponding average number of doctors per NGO was 5.4 (Table 10.5). Though, this is for an entire organization, which may be serving the entire country. However, NGO operations can be location-specific.

Fig. 10.2: NGO Type and Time of Establishment

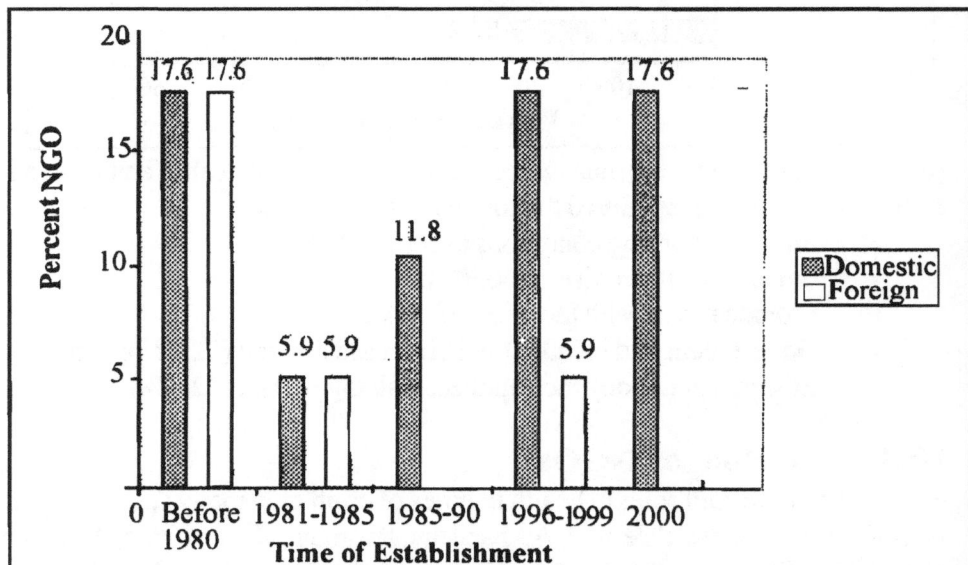

Expectedly, the supply of NGO personnel is also affected by the intensity and length of conflict. Thus, just as in the case of health facilities, the average number of staff declined with the effect of the conflict. The average number of doctors per NGO declined from 5.4 during the first year of the conflict to 5.2 during the second year of the conflict and rose to 8.4 during the first year after the conflict. This is about 62% of the average number of doctors during the second year of the conflict. This general statement can be made about all the categories of staff of the NGOs.

NGOs appear to spend a lot more than the Sierra Leonean health facilities[2]. During the second year of the conflict, for example, the average amount spent on NGO operations per organization was 6.3 million Leones, the minimum being 7.4 million Leones and the maximum, 15.1 million Leones. During the first year after the conflict, an average NGO expenditure per organization, increased to 31.8 million Leones, which is four times more than the average amount spent during the second year of the conflict. The maximum was 108 million Leones while the minimum was 12 million Leones. This suggests that NGOs appeared to contribute more to post-conflict health care in terms of the provision of funds and other resources in Sierra Leone.

Table10.5: NGO Health Staff under Conflict in Sierra Leone (Average Number)*

	1st Year Operation during Conflict	2nd Year Operation during Conflict	1st Year after Conflict
Doctors	5.4	5.2	8.4
Nurses	7.8	6.7	8.8
Pharmacists	4.5	4.1	6.4
Other Health-Professional Staff	3.1	2.8	6.4
Non-health Professional Staff	6.3	5.8	7.6
Total Health Sector Staff	27.33	24.87	35.21

*Rounding-off not done so as not to mask the changes.
Source: *Survey*

The NGO health staff that were surveyed in Sierra Leone perceived the conflict as having some inimical effects on their operations. Among these are the following:
- Staff migration/loss or layoff of staff (37.1%);
- Destruction of facilities/equipment (37.1%);
- Non-availability or high cost of drugs/expired drugs (28.6%); and
- Increased health hazard /reoccurrence of epidemics (11.4%).

NGOs working in health care in areas under conflict face a number of problems/ constraints in the pursuit of their jobs. Those identified in the survey were:
- Logistics problems (28.6%);
- Lack of security (25.7%);
- Lack of equipment/clinic/need to reconstruct damaged clinics (20.0%);
- High cost of drugs/short supply of medication (14.3%); and
- Lack of or qualified staff (11.4%).

109

10.5 Health System Performance

Many international publications rank the health system of Sierra Leone abysmally low. For the WHO *World Health Report*, 2000; using three major overall measures of good health, responsiveness to the expectations of the population, and fairness of financial contribution ranked the health system of Sierra Leone least (191st) among all the countries of the world. Using eight measures, the performance of Sierra Leone on each measure is as follows:

- Health level (Disability-Adjusted Life Expectancy—DALE): 191st;
- Health distribution: 186th;
- Responsiveness level: 173rd;
- Responsiveness distribution: 186th;
- Fairness in financial contribution: 191st;
- Overall goal attainment: 191st;
- Health expenditure per capita in international dollars: 183rd; and
- Performance on level health: 183rd.

UN (2002) also paints a gory picture about the health system performance of Sierra Leone. For example, the country had the highest infant mortality rate of 165.4 per 1000 live births in the world during the period, 1995 – 2000. Next to it is Afghanistan with 164.7. Its under-five mortality of 287.2 per 1000 live births was also the highest in the world during same period. The impact of conflict on this performance is very likely to be high. Conflict makes government not to face challenging developmental problems like education, health and eradication of poverty. Rather, hard-earned money would be spent on the acquisition of weapons and the security of the leaders.

10.6 Summary, Implications and Recommendations

The Ministry of Health and Sanitation is the only government agency in Sierra Leone that deals with health matters, whether in peace or under conflict. Its role is limited under conflict, particularly as there is no clear-cut framework of operations of health under conflict in the country. The NHP and NHAP, the two government documents on health policy in the country do not even make a passing remark about health care under conflict. Except perhaps in terms of coordination of activities of NGOs can it be seen that, the NHP gives some indirect role to government as regards post-conflict health care in its control. This is because, as was demonstrated in our analysis that NGOs make significant contributions to post-conflict health care, particularly in terms of supply of staff and funding, their coordination by a unit of the Ministry of Health and Sanitation, is therefore, indirectly, a prescribed role by the NHP. In particular, there is a need for a separate agency charged with the management of emergency situations including health. This may require developing and designing the relevant framework, promulgating adequate legislations and training the relevant human capital to address the situation.

In the area of meeting the targets set by the NHP and NHAP, the conflicts compounded the problems in Sierra Leone. The NHP painted a grim picture of the precarious health personnel situation in the country. Our analysis showed that the health personnel situation conflict was expectedly worse than peacetime situations. A salutary improvement was observable in post-conflict situations. In particular, the data collection and health information management system suffered and may account, in part, for our inability to get financial data, the monitoring activities of government including its disease surveillance as well as disease prevention and control.

In most facilities that were surveyed, the conflict began in 1991. During the period of eight to ten years that the conflict reportedly lasted, many of the facilities experienced cycles of peace and hostilities. (For example, the period included the time of the regime of Captain Valentine E. M. Strasser, later overthrown by Brigadier Biu). In the health facilities, human resources were one of those resources affected significantly by conflict. This is ably dramatized by the change in the supply of health personnel between the first year after the conflict and the second year after the conflict. Thus, the supply of doctors in the facilities during this period, increased on average by 54%, that of nurses increased by 124% while pharmacists increased by 208%. With this type of result, the proposed agency for management of emergency/conflict situations, including health, should take cognizance of such overwhelming specialized requirements in post-conflict situations, and plan for such needs *ex-ante*, perhaps using an early-warning model.

The availability of other resources in the facilities like functioning wards was also positively affected by conditions of relative peace. Thus, there was an improvement in the average number of functioning wards in post-conflict situations than under the conflict. On average, every two in three, of the surveyed facilities, were closed for at least two times during the conflict while 89% of the facilities were closed at least once. Thus, only 11% of the surveyed facilities were not shut down at all.

There were significant reductions observed in management meetings in the facilities with hostilities. That relative peace has a positive impact on the holding of management meetings is demonstrated by the fact that on average, between the first and second years after the conflict, the average number of management meetings that were held in the surveyed facilities in Sierra Leone, increased by 132%, per facility. The facilities under conflict were under stress from conflict-generated health problems. Thus, the average number of in-patients increased by 437% before the conflict and the first year of the conflict. This is not surprising, as the literature suggests that under conflict, health facility resources are diverted towards treating acute war-related health conditions.

In Sierra Leone, a significant proportion of domestic NGOs came on stream, apparently in reaction to problems posed by conflict. As many as 41.2% of the NGOs surveyed, began operations after the advent of conflict. Thus, conflict and post-conflict situations tended to encourage the influx of NGOs, particularly to address the ensuing rehabilitation problems. Our study showed that in the case of Sierra Leone, the average number of doctors per NGO during the first year after the conflict was nearly 62% more that the average number on the ground during the first year of the conflict. Also, the NGOs that were studied appear to make more significant contributions in post-conflict situations. Thus, on average, the expenditure between the first year and the second year after the conflict increased by about four times. Given the size of assistance obtained from the NGO community in Sierra Leone, it is important that their activities are effectively coordinated to avoid duplication, waste and redundancy. This will ensure that in the long run, there will be sustainable post-conflict health care delivery in the country and hence lead to the containment of the critical dilemmas of post-conflict health enunciated by Macrae (1997). This is likely to be the case under the existing situation in the country, in spite of the fact that there is an NGO coordinating unit in the Ministry of Health and Sanitation, primarily because of the huge lack of executive capacity existing in the ministry.

Given the long-drawn out nature of the conflict in Sierra Leone, the poor performance of its health system and the low health status of its peoples, during and after the conflict, it is safe to conclude that the impact of conflict on the health of the people had not been salutary. The indications are that Sierra Leone and its health system need urgent help from the international community to assist in rehabilitating its health system and the health of its peoples. This should be considered as very urgent as there is still a lot to be done.

---

[1] In general for the NGOs in Sierra Leone, missing data were observable for the year before conflict.

[2] This statement, has to be interpreted with caution since a very few facilities supplied us financial information. However, given the poor funding of health care facilities by the GOROS, it may not be too far from the true situation.

112

POTENTIALS FOR POST-CONFLICT HEALTH CARE IN NON-CONFLICT COUNTRIES AND REGIONAL INSTITUTIONS

Chapter Eleven

THE POTENTIALS FOR POST-CONFLICT HEALTH CARE IN COTE D'IVOIRE

11.1 Overview

Côte d'Ivoire, which accounts for around 70 per cent of economic production in the CFA region, witnessed considerable political instability and ethnic tension leading to loss of lives, movement of non-national residents out of the country and a downturn in the economy, in recent times. A number of people were also wounded during that period of political and social turmoil in Côte d'Ivoire. These factors created a significant risk of far larger and more complex humanitarian emergencies at the time and would continue to do so in the future.

In Côte d'Ivoire, there are general policies and procedures for the delivery of health care in emergency situations. However, there are no special policies and procedures for the delivery of health care for post conflict/emergency situations. The instruments, policies and guidelines (including laws) available to deliver health care during emergency and post conflict situations are the 'red plan' ('plan rouge') and 'ORSEC plan' ('plan ORSEC'). The 'plan rouge' is a new instrument, contained in the inter-ministerial instruction No 1279/MEMDPC/ONPC of 3rd July 2001. The objective of the Red Plan is to mitigate the consequences of an accidental or emergency situation, taking into account the following imperatives:

- The urgency of the putting into place the means of intervention;
- The rational implementation of the plan;
  The use of sufficient and appropriate means; and
- The co-ordination of the implementation of the means of medical intervention

In Cote d'Ivoire, the inter-ministerial instruction, referred to earlier, indicates that there are two government agencies designated to provide emergency health care during conflicts or other forms of emergency. These are (a) *the Service d'Aide Médicale d'Urgence* (SAMU), which means Emergency Medical Help Service and hence providing only medical services; and (b) The fire brigade, called *Groupement des Sapeurs Pompiers Militaires* (GSPM), a branch of the armed forces, which provides assistance during fire outbreaks, health emergencies and accidents.

A Prefect, called the Chief Commissioner, coordinates both the Red Plan and the ORSEC Plan. The Red Plan is implemented by a Committee headed by the Prefect and is made up of representatives of the National Office of Civil Protection (ONPC), a physician from the Urgent Medical Aid Service (SAMU), a physician from the GSPM (Military Fire Brigades Grouping), a commandant of the company (GSPM) or a commandant the State Police Force, a superintendent or a police officer. The list is not exhaustive, as the Prefect has the power to co-opt more members, if necessary, according to the requirements of the local situation.

On the other hand, the plan ORSEC was created by decree No 79-643 of 8 August 1979. ORSEC, in the final analysis, is more or less, an organization concerned with rendering assistance or help. The 'plan ORSEC' has the same objectives as the 'plan rouge'. The main objective of ORSEC is to make an inventory of, and mobilise public and private resources that can be used during floods or other disasters. They also define the conditions for their use by the authorities concerned to direct rescue.

The Red Plan is expected to be invoked when there are many victims involved in any emergency situation. The Prefect is charged with the responsibility of determining which of the two plans to invoke. He must provide the two agencies with the materials, money and other things needed to conduct the appropriate operations. He nominates the Director of Help Operations, who may be the Director of GSPM (fire brigade). He also nominates the Director of Medical Services who has to coordinate all the medical interventions in emergency situations. This could be the Director of Urgent Medical Aid Service (SAMU) or the Manager of the GSPM medical service.

During emergency situations, an advanced medical post is created outside the disaster area to administer first aid health care services. The intervention group is made up of doctors, nurses, the fire brigade and first aid workers. This group is charged with the responsibility of collecting the victims and taking them to an advanced medical post, where they will be prepared for evacuation. At the advanced medical post, a first diagnosis is made to ascertain whether an ambulance or a helicopter can evacuate them (to major public or private hospitals, and clinics). Before that, the Medical Director of SAMU must collect information from all the hospitals to determine the number of persons they can receive.

The government of Cote d'Ivoire is the major source for funding these two agencies, although supplementary funding is obtained through external assistance particularly from the European Union (European Development Fund), and the World Health Organization (WHO), among others.

Our fieldwork revealed that the two agencies require more material, human and financial resources to effectively carry out their work. In the area of material resources, they need more cars, ambulances, helicopters, technical materials, and medical consumables. In particular, the GSPM indicated that it needed at least six medical doctors and drivers. In addition, all the materials the organizations currently have are old while their equipment needs replacement. They also need money to buy or repair some of the equipment that has broken down.

To solve these problems, the agencies proposed that the Government increased their financial allocation to help them to cover their needs. The fire brigade (GSPM) indicated that in the last couple of years, it had been expecting to get additional allocation from government to pay its accumulated expenditures. In the same way, the government had to increase their human resources. To receive external assistance, the agencies would prefer direct assistance with government monitoring how the money is spent. In particular, the fire brigade would prefer to repair all its grounded equipment by creating its own internal maintenance unit. In addition, with respect to external agencies, the two local agencies propose that the Health Minister signs a form of memorandum of understanding with such external bodies to enable them assist in the event of emergencies.

11.2 Urgent Medical Aid Service (SAMU)

SAMU is a quasi-public enterprise under the Ministry of Health. Its private sector character derives from the fact that it is engaged in private sector activities for which it imposes user charges and it is also partly privately funded, particularly from the Lions' Club (provision of hospital beds, drugs and other consumables), private organisations and individuals. It has the responsibility of assuring the medical security of the people as well as seeing to the urgent evacuation/transportation of those involved in emergency situations such as accidents, fires, floods, and wars/conflicts. In the case of a massive disaster or catastrophe such as mass accidents, war/conflict, SAMU provides a special free social service, especially with respect to the vulnerable sections of the population. SAMU's services include urgent reactivation of those in coma or temporarily out of breath at home or at places of accident and other emergency situations (including 'domestic emergency'); urgently attending to those with severe burns during fire disasters (especially when privately invited or called in by GSPM); and blood cleansing in the case of insufficient renal function. Those with severe burns are usually admitted in their special hospital established for that purpose while those suffering from renal malfunction are also admitted in their special health centre established for that purpose. Apart from transporting and treating patients during emergencies ('SOS interventions') and offering the services listed above, SAMU also covers special events like football matches, attending to those who are injured in case of disasters but this is usually paid for by the match organisers. It also reinforces the activities of GSPM and the police. SAMU co-ordinates all medical interventions regarding emergency situations. It gives the first emergency health care before evacuating the victims to the nearest and the qualified health care centres by ambulance or helicopter. Its evacuation activities are to all parts of Côte d'Ivoire;

117

from Abidjan to other countries outside Africa such as those in the Americas and Europe; and to neighbouring countries. Those in need are free to dial their free call number – 185 – at anytime or other numbers such as 22 44 53 53 and 22 44 34 45.

Table 11.1 summarizes SAMU's managerial staff between 1996 and 2000, showing an increase from twelve to seventeen staff members, though between 1997 and 1999 the staff strength remained unchanged.

Table 11.1: SAMU's Managerial Staff Structure, 1996 - 2000

Managerial Staff	1996	1997	1998	1999	2000
Health Professionals	9	13	13	13	14
Health Administrative Professionals	3	3	3	3	3
Senior Executive (Total)	12	16	16	16	17
Young Supervisory Staff	-	-	-	-	-
Grand Total	12	16	16	16	17

Table 11.2 shows the fiscal allocations and the current expenditure of SAMU between 1996 and 2000. It shows that the agency ran fiscal deficits for each year for the period under consideration as allocations diverged widely from expenditure.

Table 11.2: SAMU's Fiscal Position, 1996 – 2000 (CFA)

Year	1996	1997	1998	1999	2000
Allocation	432,863,000	474,225,000	567,000,000	617,884,000	478,500,000
Current Expenditure	614,858,498	702,882,282	800,772,076	707,772,076	814,504,497

Our fieldwork indicated that SAMU had difficulties meeting its material and financial needs. As SAMU charges for its services and pays its short-term staff, if financial resources were available, it should not have human resource problems. But according to its Director, the organization has financial difficulties attending to all the cases being brought to it. With regard to material requirements, SAMU needs more vehicles, and a radio phone system to connect all the maternity hospitals. It also needs medical consumables and non-consumables. As mentioned earlier, while it is desirous of external assistance, it would prefer that such is channelled directly to it with government monitoring implementation.

11.3 *Groupment des Sapeurs Pompiers Militaires* (GSPM)

GSPM (fire brigade) is a public sector organization (a branch of the national Army) in the Ministry of Defence but under the *Chef d'état Major*. It was established by Decree No. 74-202 on 30 May 1974 but started operations on 1st July 1974. It is charged with the protection of the population and their goods against emergency threats as well as the immediate provision of emergency health services when the need arises. Being a fully public institution, residents are free to call for their services anytime, 24 hours a day, using the free call number – 180. All its services are free, unlike those of SAMU during non-catastrophic situations. GSPM has three major offices in Abidjan, Bouake, and Yamoussoukro. In Abidjan, it has three offices at Adjame, Zone 4 (Treichville), and Youpougon. GSPM has a core of operational divisions composed of a financial and administrative service, an office of employment, office of logistics, office of prevention, and office of health and social service.

GSPM examines the conditions of victims, does diagnosis and evacuates them to reference hospitals or health centres. It co-ordinates the intervention teams and the transportation of the victims, using a centre of co-ordination of operations and transport. Its operations can be categorized into three groups:

- Fire Service which involves fire of every kind including those caused by explosions or short circuits.
- Rescuing victims: discomfort/drowning/electrocution, accidents (circulation, work, household), and sanitary evacuation.
- Varied operations (research, flood, clearing of persons, menacing objects and animals, etc).

With regard to prevention, GSPM engages in the education of the populace with regard to existing rules and regulations as well as legislation; promotion of observance of security standards; visits; advice and training in enterprise; and management of fire hydrants and related activities.

Table 11.3 summarizes GSPM's managerial staff between 1996 and 2000, showing an increase from sixty-two staff members in 1996 to sixty-six in 1997. This rose to sixty -seven in 1998 before falling to fifty-four in 2000.

Table11.3: GSPM's Managerial Staff Structure, 1996 - 2000

Managerial Staff	1996	1997	1998	1999	2000
Health Professionals	41	45	46	42	36
Health Administrative Professionals	15	15	15	14	15
Senior Executive	6	6	6	5	3
Young Supervisory Staff					
Grand Total	62	66	67	61	54

Table 11.4 shows the fiscal allocations and the current expenditures of SAMU between 1996 and 2000. It shows that the GSPM, being a pure public agency, spent exactly what was allocated to it between 1996 and 1998 but in 1999 and 2000 exceeded its allocation marginally.

Table 11.4: GSPM's Fiscal Position, 1996 – 2000 (CFA)

Year	1996	1997	1998	1999	2000
Allocation	6,734,700	6,000,000	25,899,655	25,000,000	30,190,000
Current Expenditure	6,734,700	6,000,000	25,899,655	28,900,000	31,990,000

GSPM is faced with a number of problems, including inadequate human resources (it currently needs at least six medical doctors, additional nurses and drivers); and inadequate materials (especially cars and at least twenty new additional ambulances). It is faced with an acute staff shortage. It is estimated that GSPM has 931 staff to service over 16 million people currently. To make matters worse, its offices are located at far distances to the areas covered. The Abidjan offices (in the extreme South), for example, have to cover places like Korogo in the far North of the country in case of emergencies. Available equipment (such as aspirators), cars, and ambulances are very old and require replacement. Other constraints are:

- Inadequate (insufficient) implantation;
- Fall in the operating budget;
- Decrepit and insufficient materials;
- Growing operational activities; and
- Lack of physicians.

These result in excessive delay of interventions, increase in cost of operations, less driving efficiency, increased rate of unavailability, and increased dissatisfaction of the populace. The management of GSPM therefore further suggested the following:

- Decentralization of operations to increase population coverage and increased intervention efficiency.
- Greater involvement of the communes.
- Creation of rescue centres in Abidjan and in the interior of the country.
- The purchase of more operational materials for increased efficiency.

According to the management of the agency, GSPM needs 70 million franc CFA to cover the cost of emergency operations, apart from establishing an internal maintenance unit to maintain and repair their equipment.

11.4 Cross-cutting Issues

11.4.1 *Relationship between SAMU and GSPM*
At the present time, these two agencies complement one another. Thus, they work together in emergency situations. In order to handle emergencies in normal times, the SAMU hires army medical officers from GSPM and pays them. With regard to emergency situations, particularly, it's the Prefect who co-ordinates all the activities requiring emergency assistance (help).

11.4.2 *The Relationship between Government Agencies and NGOs*
There are no formal relationships between the two government agencies and the NGOs specializing in the health care delivery under emergency situations. When the services of the NGOs are required, SAMU or the Prefect gets in contact with them and enters an operational contract for mitigating the situation. The NGOs are mainly *Croix Rouge* (Red Cross) of Côte d'Ivoire, *SOS Médecins* and *Allo Docteurs*, and *l'Ordre de Malte*, which offer drugs for those admitted to hospitals/clinics.

One of the non-governmental agencies responding to the health care emergencies in the region is the International Federation of Red Cross and Red Crescent° Societies (IFRC). Its mission in West Africa is to support and encourage the West African National Red Cross and Red Crescent Societies in sixteen countries, including Côte d'Ivoire, in meeting the needs of their most vulnerable residents. Apart from carrying out relief operations to assist victims of disasters and strengthening of its member National Societies, it focuses on promoting humanitarian values, disaster response, disaster preparedness, and health and community care. With regard to health care, the focus is on:

- Improved preparation and response to epidemics;
- Reinforced awareness and prevention of HIV/AIDS;
- Support and co-ordination of West African national societies' community based first aid (CBFA) projects;
- Support to West African national societies' basic health care services; and
- Reduced incidence of female genital mutilation.

As regards disaster-mitigation preparedness, the International Federation and each National Society shall:

* Recognize that disaster preparedness should be one of the primary activities of the International Federation and each National Society, regarding it as the most effective way of reducing the impact of both small and localized as well as large-scale disasters;
* Recognize disaster preparedness as an effective link between emergency response, rehabilitation and development programmes;

121

* Recognize the Red Cross/Red Crescent role in disaster preparedness as being complementary to government and thus will not replace state responsibilities;
* Advocate, where necessary, with government, donors, non-governmental organizations and the public, the need for and effectiveness of disaster preparedness;
* Strengthen the organizational structures at international, national and local levels required for effective disaster preparedness;
* Improve co-ordination by promoting better co-operation and partnerships between National Societies, ICRC, governments, non-governmental organizations and other disaster response agencies at local, national, regional and international levels;
* Identify those persons, communities and households most at risk to disaster through assessment and analysis of risks, vulnerabilities and capacities (Vulnerability and Capacity Assessment) as a basis for prioritizing location and focusing of programming activities;
* Raise awareness of disaster hazards through public education, encouraging vulnerable people to take preventative and mitigating actions where possible before disaster strikes;
* Improve the ability of vulnerable communities to cope with disasters through community-based disaster preparedness strategies that build on existing structures, practices, skills and coping mechanisms; and
* Strive to provide the financial, material and human resources required to carry out appropriate and sustainable disaster preparedness activities.

With regard to disaster emergency response, the International Federation and each National Society shall:
* Seek to assist the most vulnerable people in emergencies. (These encompass at a minimum, adequate safe water and sanitation, adequate food, adequate health care including psychological support and adequate shelter);
* Recognize the Red Cross and Red Crescent role as auxiliary to government in humanitarian activities;
* Undertake emergency response according to the Fundamental Principles of the Red Cross and Red Crescent;
* Work within the competence of the Operating National;
* Base their actions on appropriate disaster preparedness programming and planning;
* Work towards self-reliance and sustainability of programming;
* Continue until the acute threat to life and health has abated; and
* Maximize the strategic advantage of the International Federation by 'working as a Federation' to mobilize all appropriate resources.

Post-emergency rehabilitation activities are also undertaken with the active participation of the community in the planning and implementation of the activities on the basis of a timely and thorough assessment of unmet needs and available response capacity. Should assistance be given, it ensures that it is targeted to the most needy and most vulnerable groups and complements rather than replaces the responsibilities and activities of government services.

The Red Cross of Côte d'Ivoire (RCCI) was founded in 1960 and joined the Movement in 1963. The statutes and rules of procedure were amended at the last general assembly, held in March 1996. It is autonomous and independent, but its relationship with the government is not sufficiently defined. There are thirty-five local committees, principally a central committee and a steering committee. The society has twelve salaried members of staff. At the committee level, there are no paid staff; the committees are run exclusively by volunteers. Out of a total volunteer base of approximately 7,800, there are around 1,000 young volunteers. Volunteers are an important resource, having gained experience through the Liberian refugee operation. The RCCI makes use of volunteers in its first-aid and awareness activities and co-operates with the government and UN agencies in the field of assistance to refugees. The society is also a member of the national planning committee for the national disaster preparedness plan and regional health plan.

In addition to support from the International Federation and the ICRC, external assistance has been received from the Netherlands, and British and Spanish Red Cross Societies for community health, institutional development and programmes assisting vulnerable children. In 1998, for example, the RCCI's expenditure totalled approximately 1.3 million F CFA. Domestic income accounts for around 20 per cent of the budget, while funding from external partners provides the remaining 80 per cent.

The RCCI's domestic income comes from its membership and from two schools it operates. It receives the modest sum of 12,200 F CFA from the communes each year. The largest source of income is the Movement. Some income-generating activities are carried out, and the society recognizes that this is an area, which it needs to strengthen, together with improvements in financial management. The RCCI's property includes its headquarters with a kindergarten, a primary school and a nutrition centre. In 1998, the society acquired a centre for first-aid training. Most local branch committees do not have their own building, which sometimes hinders their activities. The society owns seven vehicles, three of which were provided for the Liberian refugee operation.

The RCCI opened a clinic for people injured in the post-election violence in October 2000. The clinic is located in Adjame, a neighbourhood adjacent to the central administrative district, Le Plateau. Adjame and other low-income neighbourhoods such as Abobo, Anyama and Youpougon saw much of the unrest on 25-26 October that followed a call for new elections by the opposition *Rassemblement des Republicains* (RDR) party. Scores of people died while hundreds of others were wounded. Some were treated under tents outside the home of RDR leader, Alassane Ouattara.

After violence broke out again in Abidjan on 4th December, 2000, the Red Cross mobilised its first-aid teams and delivered medical supplies to the five main hospitals of the economic capital of Côte d'Ivoire. With the help of the ICRC and the International Federation of Red Cross and Red Crescent Societies, the Red Cross Society of Côte d'Ivoire deployed 124 first-aid workers to provide emergency relief to the country's main cities (Abidjan, Bouaké, Gagnoa, Divo and Odienné) until the legislative elections were held. In Abidjan, where most of the clashes took place, eight teams gave first aid to the wounded and evacuated them to hospitals. According to estimates, a total of 256 wounded people were treated on 4th, 5th and 6th December 2000. On 4th and 5th December, 2000 the ICRC also distributed medical supplies to Cocody, Treichville, Abobo and Yopougon hospitals. Those supplies were to make it possible to treat 350 wounded. Also, after approaching the authorities on 6th December, 2000, the ICRC was given access to the people arrested during the violence and hence was able to visit 328 people detained in Abidjan to determine their health care needs and provide them.

11.5 Recent Experiences on Refugee Situations and Emergency Operations in Côte d'Ivoire

By 1998, there were about 350,000 Liberian refugees in Côte d'Ivoire. According to UNHCR, in 2000 there were 110,000 Liberian refugees in Côte d'Ivoire, of which some 50,000 remain unregistered. There were also about 2,000 Sierra Leonean refugees on the Western borders. There was concern that deterioration in either the internal security of Côte d'Ivoire or in the sub region as a whole may force an unplanned return of over 100,000 refugees to their country of origin.

However, in 2001, instability in neighbouring Guinea and fighting in the Lofa region of Liberia has brought in a new influx of refugees into Cote d'Ivoire. According to UNHCR, there were 120,000, mostly Liberian refugees, left after an influx in 1999. A recent update reported that a steady flow of fifty Liberian refugees a day has been entering Côte d'Ivoire since early May 2001 when fighting broke out in Lofa county, northern Liberia.

The refugees were accommodated in the *Zone d'Accueil des Refugies* (ZAR). which is an area designated by the Ivorian government to shelter refugees. The ZAR is made up of two prefectures, Danane, located only 30 km from Liberia, and Guiglo, 150 km to the south of Danane and the refugees are not permitted to move outside this area. Guiglo contains the only refugee camp in Côte d'Ivoire, called Nicla, which currently has a population of 8,000 people. The rest of the refugee population lives in parts of Guiglo and Danane and ten small towns in between. Reports of the new refugee influx have indicated that most appear to be girls and women between five and sixty years of age. The high proportion of women and children make the new refugees particularly vulnerable as a result of poor work opportunities, and the population is likely to be dependent on humanitarian assistance for the immediate future. The World Food Programme has begun distributions to 500 newly arrived refugees who have already arrived in Nicla camp in Guiglo. The 500 are the initial caseload out of 1,068 who registered to go to the camp.

Currently, many of the long-term refugees in Côte d'Ivoire receive assistance and are able to seek employment and are therefore not considered at high risk. However, the new refugees are likely to be at slightly elevated risk as a result of their recent displacement and the high percentage of women and children in the population. Their situation will need careful monitoring.

Some recommended measures to improve the situation include:
* Improving surveillance systems for both nutrition and health at the local level.
* Ensuring that contingency planning has been done for the health and nutrition sectors.

11.6   Conclusion

In Cote d'Ivoire, health care delivery under conflict/emergency situations rests with the two government agencies of SAMU and GSPM as well as NGOs typified by the Red Cross Society of Cote d'Ivoire. The analysis in this section suggests the existence of a fairly comfortable institutional infrastructure in terms of the rules and regulations, legislations, and a network of identifiable organizations for health care delivery under conflict even up to the community level. There is also a clear recognition of the roles of NGOs in health care delivery under conflict, disaster-mitigation preparedness and disaster/emergency response. However, there is a grave limitation to the extent of reach of the activities of these organizations being located very far from most parts of the country, as well as limited financial, material (particularly equipment and logistics) and human resources. Worthy of note is that, the country, though not under conflict has more experience than most non-conflict West African countries in refugee and conflict management, in general, and health care delivery under conflict, in particular, because of the influx of refugees from the conflict countries of Liberia and Sierra Leone and the spill-over of Sierra Leonean and Liberian refugees from the Republic of Guinea.

However, in spite of the strong tradition for collaboration between the government and NGOs in disaster mitigation and emergency care in the country, there is no indication that there is a strong unit that can effectively coordinate the activities of NGOs, particularly NNGOs, to contain problems of duplication of activities as well as wastage and redundancies in health care delivery under conflict and in post-conflict situations. Consequently, it may be difficult, under existing situations, to contain the critical dilemmas of post conflict health rehabilitation (Macrae, 1997) in Cote d'Ivoire if the necessary institutional and legal framework is not in place. This study suggests that this be done.

Chapter Twelve

THE POTENTIALS FOR POST-CONFLICT HEALTH CARE IN NIGERIA

12.1 Introduction

Since independence in 1960, Nigeria has fought a civil war (1967- 70), experienced a number of ethno-religious and other communal crises as well as major disasters like the air disaster of September 19, 1992 involving a military plane in which about 163 senior military officers lost their lives; the air crash of ADC flight 086 near Ejinrin, Epe in Lagos State in which 144 passengers died and the bomb blast of January 2002 in Ikeja Military Cantonment with its attendant high toll of human and material losses estimated to cost several billions of Naira.

There have been other numerous disasters like fire outbreaks, kerosene and pipeline explosions etc; all over the political landscape in recent times. In all these occasions, the impotence of the nation's conflict/emergency management agencies was laid bare. Given this situation, there are bound to be questions on the state of preparedness of the nation to mitigate future conflicts and emergencies especially as it relates to the health of victims of the various conflict situations and disasters.

In this section of the study, we assess the existing policies, guidelines instruments and institutions available in the country to mitigate conflicts/emergencies generally, and the post-conflict/emergency health care delivery situation, in particular.

12.2 Overview

Various attempts have been made in Nigeria since independence in 1960, to modify post-conflict/emergency situations. The first major attempt was the establishment of the Nigerian Red Cross Society (NRCS) through an Act of Parliament in 1960, and its incorporation in 1961. Initially the NRCS was mandated to assist the distressed and wounded wherever found, without discrimination. At that time the NRCS, was more or less, ancillary to government in the areas of disaster, health and social welfare. However, its functions expanded in scope over the years, as will be seen later.

After NRCS, the National Committee on Ecological Problems, mandated to check desertification by embarking on tree planting, was established. It was basically funded from the Ecological Fund, set aside by the Federal Government to confront problems posed by environmental degradation of various types and funded annually to the tune of 2% of the federation account. In reaction to the toxic waste dump at Koko, a town in Bendel State now consisting of Edo and Delta States, the Waste Disposal Decree of 1988 was promulgated and this metamorphosed later into the Federal Environmental Protection Agency Decree of March 29 1989.

Increased road mishaps in Nigeria, with the attendant gruesome causalities, led to another attempt at mitigating disasters from emanating road accidents, subsequently, through the Federal Road Safety Act Cap 141, the Federal Road Safety Corps (FRSC) came into being. Its mandate includes preventing accident-related disasters through the policing of the highways, setting driving standards, rescuing accident victims, among others. The FRSC was merged with the Nigeria Police under the military. However, under the new civilian regime, it has regained its independence.

Due to the inadequacies of existing government agencies to handle the emergency situations at the end of the Nigerian civil war (1967-1970) in January 1970, there came the need to establish an appropriate institutional framework to take care of the needs of several hundreds of thousands of war victims. Accordingly, Decree 48 of 1976 was promulgated to establish an agency with the mandate of providing relief for, and engage in the rehabilitation of civil war victims. On board came a new agency, known as the National Emergency Relief Agency (NERA), which was, as its name suggests, basically relief-oriented.

As urbanization and industrialization increased, natural and human-activity-induced disasters multiplied. Global warming, increased desertification, deforestation, landslides, fire outbreaks and explosions, increased politically fanned ethnic clashes resulting in thousands of causalities, collapsed buildings arising from structural defects and low standards of construction materials, etc are some of the disasters that grew with Nigeria's development. Some government parastatals/departments like the Nigeria Police Force, Nigeria Armed Forces, The Nigeria Fire Service, and some Non-Governmental Organizations (NGOs), are all stakeholders in the conflict/ emergency management in the country. The NERA, however, is the foremost among these stakeholders in terms of capital and human resources, investment and commitment to disaster management in the country. NERA became incapable of handling these situations because of several factors such as limited instruments, policy guidelines, inadequate human and capital resources, etc.

The National Emergency Management Agency (NEMA) is the metamorphosis of NERA vides Decree 12 of 23rd March 1999. No doubt, the establishment of NEMA marked the first major attempt at comprehensively addressing problems arising from conflict and emergency situations in Nigeria. A number of policy guidelines and instruments have been developed over time for its operations. If these are fully implemented, many of the pressing issues thrown up by the many conflict/emergency situations plaguing the country, will be effectively tackled. However, as it will be seen in our subsequent analysis, there is still a lot to be done, particularly in the area of health care delivery under conflict/ emergencies

12.3 Existing Instruments and Agencies For Conflict/ Emergency Management

The basic instrument established to effectively manage conflict/emergency situations came into being on March 25 1999 through Decree 12 of the Federal Republic of Nigeria. The decree in part 1(i) established a body known as the *National Emergency Management Agency* (NEMA) as a corporate body with perpetual succession; which can sue and be sued in its corporate name. The decree also established a Governing Council for NEMA, which has as its chairman, the nation's Vice President. Among its members are the Secretary to the Government of the Federation, a representative, not below the rank of a Director from each of seven Federal Ministries: Aviation, Foreign Affairs, Health, Internal Affairs, Transport, Water Resources, and Works and Housing. Other members of the NEMA Governing Council are representatives of the armed forces, the police, the Nigerian Red Cross Society and such voluntary organizations that may be determined from time to time. The functions of NEMA, spelt out in Part II of the decree establishing it include:

- Formulation of policy on disaster management, coordination of plans, strategies, programmes for efficient and effective response to disasters at national level.
- Coordination and promotion of research in disaster management.
- Monitoring the state of preparedness of all stakeholders that contribute to disaster management.
- Procurement, receipt of donations and distribution of emergency relief materials to victims of disasters and to also assist in rehabilitation work where necessary, etc.

The decree establishing NEMA defines *natural and other disasters*, which the agency is set up to manage very broadly to include 'any disaster arising from any crisis, epidemic, drought, flood, earthquake, storm, train, roads, aircraft, oil spillage or other accidents and mass deportation or repatriation of Nigerians from any other country' (section 6(2)). Given this broad definition and the membership of the Governing Council of NEMA, the subject matter of this study can be seen to fall within the purview of this agency. The extent to which this is true in practice will be revealed by our subsequent analysis.

NEMA is saddled with the responsibility of coordinating the activities of all disaster management bodies such as, the International Red Cross and Red Crescent Society (IRCS), Nigeria Red Cross and Red Crescent Society (NRCS), local NGOs and community-based organizations (CBOs), the organized private sector (construction consortiums like Julius Berger, big oil companies like Chevron Oil or

Shell Petroleum Development Company, etc,), Military and Paramilitary agencies, etc. The decree establishing NEMA also made provision for each state of the Federation to set up a State Emergency Management Committee with spelt-out functions which include; notification of the apex agency (NEMA) of any natural or other disasters occurring within the state, responding to disasters and seeking for assistance from NEMA where necessary, etc. (Part III 9 (a) – (d) of the decree). The decree also provides for funding the agency through:

(a) Allocation from the Federation Account;
(b) 20% of the 2% of the Ecological Fund;
(c) Grants from Federal, or State or Local Governments;
(d) Grants from the organized private sector, international or donor organizations and NGOs;
(e) Gifts, loans, grants –in- aid, testamentary disposition or otherwise; and
(f) All monies received from the National Emergency Trust Fund, and all other assets accruing to the agency.

NEMA's operational concept is tailored towards achieving an effective and efficient disaster management. Its structure depicts four distinct departments to address Pre-disaster Management, Point of Contact Management and Post Disaster Management. The four departments are:

(i) The Planning, Research and Forecasting;
(ii) Search, Rescue and Disaster Prevention;
(iii) Relief and Rehabilitation; and
(iv) Finance and Administration (Figure 12. 1)

Figure 12.1: National Emergency Management Agency Organizational Chart

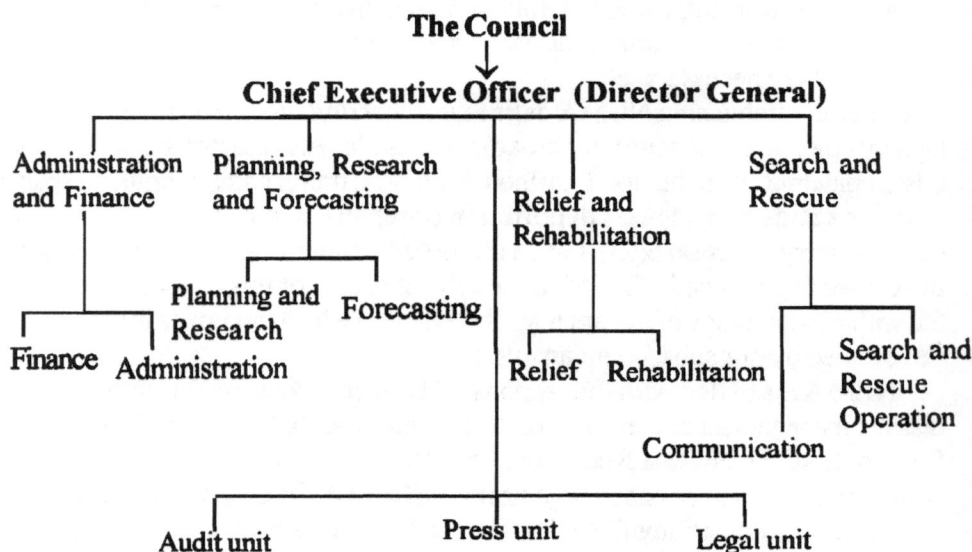

(i) **Planning, Research and Forecasting Department**

The Department of Planning, Research and Forecasting is responsible for the planning of all activities of NEMA both internally and externally. It also ensures effective plan implementation and evaluation. This department is expected to come up with disaster/risk maps, which could assist in preparedness planning, emergency responses and early warning. When fully operational, thisdepartment is expected to substantially prop up public awareness of natural and man-induced hazards, and to reduce risks (loss of life, social and economic costs, etc) occasioned by hazards.

(ii) **The Department of Search, Rescue and Disaster Prevention**

It is the interventionist organ that responds to disaster occurrence especially when such situations exceed the capability of local/state government. It conducts emergency operations to save lives and property. The department has a Disaster Reaction Unit headed by a serving Wing Commander in the Nigerian Air force, which when fully operational, is expected to respond faster to distress calls/emergency situations. The Federal Executive Council has approved the Unit's 'COSPAS-SARSAT' programme for the notification of marine and aircraft distress messages across the country. As quick response units, they are the nation's arrowhead for the prevention of situations leading to marine/aircraft emergency calls (as in the case of terrorism, for example), and are legally bound to react to them when they occur.

While not having a full-blown medical outfit, the department has some health professionals including physiotherapists and psychologists that can offer urgent post-conflict medical services to victims. NEMA is mandated to call on the Federal Ministry of Health, Specialist Hospitals, all Health Organizations, other medical NGOs and the Nigerian Red Cross Society to respond to health issues in times of emergencies.

NEMA also has some basic medical equipment at its disposal to handle some situations e.g. ambulance services, water purification tankers to ensure clean and potable water supply in emergency situations; extricating instruments for use in cases of accident victims; body bags for decomposing bodies to stem epidemic outbreak, etc. The department plans to have a working relationship with professional bodies such as the Nigerian Society of Engineers (NSE) and Council of Registered Engineers of Nigeria (COREN) to ensure that building standards are not compromised on thereby forestalling or minimizing collapsed-structures related disasters.

(iii) **The Department of Relief and Rehabilitation**

The department attends to the basic needs of disaster/conflict victims in terms of the provision of food, shelter, water, medical care and the restoration of essential public utilities. The department's mandate also includes data-banking relief materials sources in collaboration with other departments especially that of Planning, Research and Forecasting. It is also charged with the keeping of stock of relief materials and identifying sources of monetary donations.

The Relief, and Rehabilitation department is in close collaboration with the NRCS, which has much longer standing and coverage in this field (the total number of volunteers of the IRCS as at 2001 is estimated at 105 million worldwide). It has a total of 250,000 volunteers in Nigeria alone.

The department also works in close collaboration with other NGOs in Disaster Management. The relief and rehabilitation work of the agency is not limited to the shores of Nigeria alone; but extends to other African nations like Chad, Niger, Liberia, etc.

(iv) Department of Finance and Administration

The department co-ordinates the day to day administration and finances of the agency. The administrative unit ensures that productivity and efficiency are the personnel's watchword. The finance unit liaises with the Federal Ministry of Finance (FMF), the Accountant General's office, other ministries and the office of the Vice President for effective and prudent financial resource management. Its main source of fund is the accrual to the agency through the 20% of the 2% National Ecological Fund.

With these structures on the ground already, and a close evaluation of the activities of the agency (NEMA) since its inception in 1999, it has come a long way in attempting to achieve its mandates, as entrenched in the decree establishing it.

In general, in Nigeria, there are multiple agencies responsible for health care delivery under conflict/ emergency situations. They can be categorized into five groups:

(a) The Emergency preparedness and response Unit of the Federal Ministry of Health.

(b) All the Federal Hospitals (government owned) in all the states of the country (36 states) and the Federal Capital Territory (FCT) Abuja.

(c) All Teaching/Specialist Hospitals and the Federal Medical Centres.

(d) All Local Government Health Offices in Nigeria and the Nigerian Red Crescent/Red Cross Society.

(e) The National Emergency Management Agency (NEMA) under part II section 6.1 subsection (0) is involved in post- conflict/emergency health care delivery. The subsection states that NEMA shall 'perform such others functions which in the opinion of the Agency are required for the purpose of achieving its objective under this decree'.

(a) **The Federal Ministry of Health:** Apart from the main function of formulating policies and guidelines and providing support to lower tiers of government, the ministry also heads a National Committee on Emergency Preparedness and Response which the Honourable Minister of Health chairs. The National Committee on Emergency Preparedness and Response has membership drawn from international bodies like the World Health Organization (WHO), United Nations Children's Fund (UNICEF); NGOs like the Red Cross and Red Crescent Society, etc.

(b) **The General Hospitals, Teaching and Specialist Hospitals and the Federal Medical Centres:** They are all responsible for the management of health cases arising from conflicts and emergencies. They are to manage the cases with a view of ameliorating the suffering of the victims and to control outbreaks of diseases affecting victims or that might result from the conflicts/disasters. These institutions are responsible for health care management without discrimination in conflict and emergency situations especially those resulting from fire, accident and blasts to ensure that victims' lives are saved.

(c) **The Local Government Health Offices, Nigeria Red Cross and Red Crescent Society and other NGOs:** The health care departments at the third tier of government and NGOs like the Nigeria Red Cross and Red Crescent Society (NRCS) are mainly charged with advocacy and social mobilization. The Local Health Centres are to respond to emergency cases even at first aid level in conflicts/ emergencies arising within their area of jurisdiction and to seek for assistance from health institutions operating at higher levels of health care delivery or make referrals as the situation dictates. However, the NRCS, through its numerous activities has transcended mobilization and advocacy to make inroads, in some instances, to health care delivery in emergency, post-emergency and post-conflict cases.

Though, its initial mandate was to be an ancillary to the National Government in matters relating to disaster, health and social welfare, in recent times, it has become more concerned with the alleviation of human suffering especially the most vulnerable in conflict/disaster situation: the women, children, aged and the disabled. Basically, its sole aim is total commitment to the alleviation of human suffering and the protection of human life and dignity.

Specifically, the society has been involved in the distribution of relief materials, rehabilitation, first aid services and psychological support services; maternal and child health care delivery through the mother clubs; medical care and counselling for people living with AIDS (PLWA), immunization, prison health programme; highway ambulance services, family reunion (a post emergency/ conflict programme), etc.

133

There are a few indigenous NGOs in the area of emergency care. Perhaps, foremost amongst them is the African Refugee Foundation (AREF), which was established in 1994 by Ambassador Segun Olusola in response to the overwhelming demands of the Rwandan genocide by the majority Hutu population on the minority Tutsi ethnic group or their Hutu sympathizers. AREF has been involved in complex emergencies and disasters in many African countries like Ethiopia, Eritrea, Burundi, etc. It was involved in health care delivery under conflict in the horn of Africa in collaboration with *Doctors for all Nations* by providing non-prescription medicines and other supplies. AREF is said to have its own corps of medical and health volunteers who can be mobilized and allocated to areas of conflict at very short notice. In spite of this promise, AREF still has limitations in the area of health care delivery under conflict; it needs more formal and careful planning in this regard. It has also collaborated with LASU to establish a research centre in peace and conflict studies and to build capacity for conflict resolution and management through a diploma course in peace and conflict studies.
However, this does not contain formal training in health care delivery under conflict/emergency situations.

(d) **National Emergency Management Agency:** The National Emergency Management Agency is the chief coordinator of all Emergency/Conflict Management stakeholders in Nigeria. Due to its relative early start and considering the enormous task in its kitty, coupled with its present manpower resources and capacity-building limitations, it appears not to have given the issue of post- conflict/emergency health care delivery, the attention it needs. However, the overall co-ordination of post conflict/emergency management generally, the health sector inclusive, is the responsibility of NEMA as stipulated in the decree establishing it; but coordination of health issues including those with conflict/emergencies implications fall within the purview of the Federal Ministry of Health. Thus, there is an intersection of responsibilities as regards health care delivery under conflict/emergency activities, in the functions of NEMA and the Federal Ministry of Health. Besides, there are a number of agencies through which NEMA implements its plans, including those relating to health care delivery. It does this, as will be seen from its National Disaster Response Plan (NDRP), discussed later in this section, through signed letters of agreement indicating commitment to partnerships for addressing problems of emergency/disaster management.

The evolution of NEMA as the main government agency responsible for emergency/ relief management in Nigeria from 1960 at independence to date can be categorized into five phases based on the organizational leadership.

- The first phase of the National Council for Rehabilitation (1960 –1976), when the concern was mainly relief-focused and under the leadership of Timothy Onobare;
- The brief leadership of S. C. Nwokoche of the National Emergency Relief (NERA) in 1976;
- The NERA period 1976 – 1992 under the old guidelines;
- The NERA revival period under the 1993 guidelines which lasted till 1995 and under the leadership of J. A. A. Alibaloye; and
- The National Emergency Management Agency Period from 1995 under the leadership of Mrs Oluremi Olowu.

There are no data on the staff situation of the government agency responsible for conflict/disaster management in the early days. From 1976, however, the total staff strength, varied between fifty-four to eighty during the period 1976-1992 and eighty-five in 1993 (Table 12.2). From the days of NEMA, the staff strength rose dramatically to 118 in 1995 for example. It rose further to 127 in 1996 but dropped to 111 in 1997 and further to eighty-seven and eighty-two in 1998 and 1999, respectively. It rose by nearly 50% to 121 in 2000 and marginally to 134 in 2001. Clearly, the availability of staff in the right quality, skill composition and number can be seen to be a major constraint of this agency.

Table 12.1: Human Resources of Government Institutions Charged with Conflict/Emergency Management 1960-1993

Year	Organisation	Junior Staff	Senior Staff	Total
1960-1976	National Council for Rehabilitation headed by Chief Timothy Onobare	Not Available	Not Available	
1976	NERA headed by Mr S. C Nwokoche	50	4	54
1976-1992	NERA	Varied	Between 54 and 80	In total
1993	NERA Amendment Act 113 headed by Mr Alibaloye J.A.A	77	8	85

Source: *Field Work*

Table 12.2: Human Resources of the National Emergency Management Agency 1995– 2001

Year	Junior Staff	Senior Staff	Total
1995	82	36	118
1996	92	35	127
1997	76	35	111
1998	58	29	87
1999	54	28	82
2000	68	53	121
2001	79	55	134

Source: *NEMA Abuja Field Work*

(v)   The National Disaster Response Plan

The National Disaster Response Plan (NDRP), is an operations-oriented document authorized by NEMA, which describes the mechanism by which the Federal Government mobilizes resources and conducts activities aimed at addressing the consequences of any major disaster or emergency that overwhelms the capacity of state and local governments in the country (NEMA, 2001).

To carry out the activities specified in the NDRP, NEMA, through signed letters of agreement, cooperates with a number of Federal Ministries, departments and agencies.

The letter of agreement commits the organization to:

- support the NDRP concept of operations and carry out the assigned functional responsibilities to ensure the orderly, timely delivery of federal assistance;
- cooperate with NEMA to provide effective oversight of disaster operations;
- make maximum use of existing authorities, organizations, resources, systems, and programmes to reduce disaster relief costs;
- form partnerships with counterpart state agencies, voluntary disaster relief organizations, and the private sector to take advantage of existing resources; and
- continue to develop and refine headquarters and zonal planning, exercise, and training activities to maintain necessary operational capabilities.

The signatories to this agreement are the Federal Ministry of Aviation, the Federal Ministry of Health, the Federal Ministry of Transport, the Federal

Ministry of Works and Housing, Federal Ministry of Agriculture, Ministry of Power and Steel, Ministry of Foreign Affairs, Ministry of Internal Affairs, Ministry of Water Resources, Federal Ministry of Finance, Ministry of Environment, Nigerian National Petroleum Corporation, National Electric Power Authority, Defence Headquarters, Nigeria Police, Nigerian Red Cross Society and NEMA.

The NDRP supports the implementation of the NEMA Act as amended, as well as other individual agency statutory authorities. It also supplements other federal emergency plans developed to address specific hazards. *Inter alia*, the NDRP:

- sets forth fundamental policies, planning assumptions, a concept of operations, response, and recovery actions, and federal agency and private sector responsibilities;
- describes the array of federal response, recovery, and mitigation resources available to augment state and local efforts to save lives; protect public health, safety, and property;
- organizes the forms of federal response assistance that a state is most likely to require under thirteen support service areas (SSAs); each of which has a designated primary agency;
- spells out the processes and methodology for implementing and managing federal recovery and mitigation programmes and support/technical services;
- provides a focus for interagency and intergovernmental emergency preparedness, planning, training, exercising, coordinating, and information exchange; and
- serves as the foundation for the development of detailed supplemental plans and procedures to implement federal response and recovery activities rapidly and efficiently.

In terms of scope, the NDRP applies only to such situations that qualify to be described as major disasters or emergencies, which include natural catastrophes; fire, flood or explosion regardless of cause; or any other occasion or instance for which the President determines that federal assistance is needed to supplement state and local efforts and capabilities.

Its activities cover a full range of complex and constantly changing requirements following a disaster: saving lives, protecting property, and meeting basic human needs (response); restoring the disaster-affected area (recovery); and reducing vulnerability to future disasters (mitigation). However, it does not address long-term reconstruction and development.

The NDRP is made up of three parts:

- The basic plan, which presents the policies and concepts of operations that guide how the Federal Government will assist disaster-stricken states and local governments. It also summarizes federal planning assumptions, response and recovery actions.

- Support Services Areas (SSAs) section, which describes the mission, policies, concept of operations, and responsibilities of the primary and support agencies involved in the implementation of the key response functions that supplement state and local activities. SSAs include Transport, Communications, Public Works and Engineering, Firefighting, Information and Planning, Mass Care, Resource Support, Health and Medical Services, Search and Rescue, Hazardous Materials, Food, Energy and Military/Police Support.
- The Recovery Function section describes the policies, planning considerations, and concept of operations that guide the provision of assistance to help disaster victims and the affected communities return to normal life and minimize the risk of future damage. Assistance given is categorized by delivery system—either to individuals, families, and businesses or to states and local governments.

In its hazard analysis, the NDRP asserts that Nigeria is vulnerable to hazards, which it groups into natural and man-made hazards. Identified as natural disasters are: flooding, coastal erosion, gully erosion, drought, wildfire, sand storm, thunderstorm and wind storm, pest invasion; and volcanic eruption and associated activities. Classified as man-made disasters are civil disturbances, particularly riots and demonstrations, dam failure, mine pit collapse, building collapse, oil spillage, maritime disasters, air accidents, bomb blast, road accidents, train accidents, fire accidents; and hazardous material spillage/dangerous cargo.

The NDRP is a comprehensive document. It contains important information, including addresses and telephone numbers of the agencies and officials to contact in the event of any disaster. Among such agencies and/or officials are NEMA (with emergency hot lines specified); the three arms of the armed forces; in particular, the Nigerian Army and the Nigerian Air Force Disaster Response Units; the Federal Road Safety Corps; the Federal and State Fire Services; the officials of the FMOH to contact in the event of any epidemic outbreak; the state command of the Nigeria Security and Civil Defence Corps; and the list of government hospitals, by state.

Thus, with the way the NDRP is designed and formulated, it has the potential for being adapted for health care delivery under conflict and in post-conflict situations. It is quite comprehensive and integrated, with health care being just a part of the disaster management. However, it focused *mainly* on the short-term end of the relief-rehabilitation-development continuum.

(vi)   The National Commission for Refugees (NCFR)

The NCFR was established under Decree 59 of 1989 (Cap 244 Law of the Federation of Nigeria, 1990) and is the main instrument for the protection and management of refugees in Nigeria. The law is a follow-up to the 1951 Geneva Convention, the 1967 Protocol and the 1969 OAU Convention governing specific aspects of refugee problems in Africa. The Act is meant to conform with, and accelerate the efforts at the international and regional levels aimed at solving the numerous problems facing people seeking refugee status outside their countries of origin as a result of war, persecution on grounds of race, religion, etc (Ogbaji, 2003).

Generally, the NCFR is concerned with refugees who are victims of war and other internal conflicts particularly in the West African subregion. As a result of the perennial crisis in the subregion, in the last decade or so, national refugee camps were set up in Oru, Ogun State and Maiduguri, Borno State. The management of the camp inmates is a collaborative work between the NCFR, NGOs and international donor agencies such as Caritas, UNICEF and the IRCS etc (Olusola, 2003). Besides, in 2001, over 200 Liberian refugees were admitted en block to Nigeria on account of the renewed hostilities in that country, on the orders of the President. Nigeria is also expecting as many as 5,000 refugees to relocate to Nigeria from Cote d'Ivoire on account of the recent disturbances resulting from renewed hostilities there (Ogbaji, 2003).

With the dramatic increase in communal violence in Nigeria, since the return of civilian rule in 1999, nearly all parts of the country have been plunged into a number of conflicts which are classified mainly as indigene-settler conflicts; inter-ethnic or intra-ethnic conflicts; intra- or inter-political party conflicts, and religious conflicts. This has increased the phenomenon of internally displaced persons (IDPs) in Nigeria to well over 750,000 in 2003. Accordingly, the original mandate of the commission, which concerns mainly the welfare of refugees was expanded to incorporate the welfare of IDPs (Olusola, 2003).

Olusola (2003) reported that the NCFR, in consultation with other stakeholders, has designed a comprehensive welfare package in the form of self-employment schemes for inmates of the national refugee camps. The schemes are basically to enable the inmates acquire different skills in areas that will be beneficial to them.

It can be seen that the NCFR, focuses on the medium to long-term end of the relief-rehabilitation-development continuum. However, there is no formal recognition for the role of the organization in health care delivery under conflict or in post-conflict situations. This needs to be given the formal recognition it deserves.

139

12.4   Constraints and Limitations

Nigeria could be said to be generally bereft of any *planned* or *organized* quick response apparatus on which she could fall back in times of emergency, before the emergence of NEMA. NERA, the agency that existed earlier, was generally inefficient, ill-equipped and under-funded. Since the inception of NEMA, however, and judging from the management of recent conflicts and disasters across the country, there has been some improvement, in terms of response, particularly in the area of relief. Rescue and rehabilitation responses still lag behind. One of the major problems facing organizations charged with disaster management is a gross lack of funds. In 2002, the Honourable Minister for Works and Housing admitted that the Federal Fire Service needs as much as ₦4.6 billion to put it in proper shape i.e. effective and functional. Activities of most NGOs involved in disaster management especially as regards rescue and responses are also hampered by inadequate funds. The Nigeria Red Cross Society seems to fare better because of financial and logistic support it receives from the IRCS.

The financial losses recorded during the January 27th 2002 bomb blast in Lagos was put at several hundreds of billions of Naira. Meanwhile, many conflicts and disasters that occur across the country all beg for attention in the face of the meagre allocation from the federation account to the sole agency saddled with the responsibility of disaster/conflict management.

Even when funds are made available, co-ordination between stakeholders in disaster management, especially in response and rescue, is inefficient and ineffective. There was the case in May 2002 when the warehouse of NEMA in Lagos went up in flames. Improper coordination resulted in insufficient water supply that rendered the ill- equipped (in terms of vehicular strength and manpower) fire service impotent; thereby allowing relief materials worth millions of Naira to be gutted by fire. The effective coordination and networking mandate of NEMA can only be achieved when it is properly funded, monitored and evaluated, albeit periodically.

There is also the problem of ignorance on the part of the populace. The population's response to disasters, calls for greater public enlightenment campaigns and mobilization.

The commitment and sincerity of various tiers of government, especially the federal government, poses a bottleneck to effective conflict/emergency management. Due to incessant changes in the administration of the country in the past years, government policies and guidelines were never continuous or stable. While some governments see conflict/disaster management purely from a relief point of view, others perceive it purely from the rehabilitation viewpoint. This narrow focus inhibits development and affects broader issues like post-conflict health delivery, the focus of this study, adversely.

There is also the logistics problem in disaster/conflict management in Nigeria. The requisite equipment, which is necessary for effective response and rescue, are not in place. For instance, effective communication gadgets, warning/alert signals, disaster forecasting tools, like early-warning models, etc are lacking. However, the situation has improved slightly with the recent GSM revolution in Nigeria.

Inadequate capacity building and training in anticipation of conflict/disaster situations is totally absent in the country. A case in point is the January 2002 bomb blast in Lagos, which resulted in the drowning of many of the victims in canals. It was impossible to get professional divers to assist in the rescue operation because the country apparently has little or none of them at all. Rather, local fishermen were credited for the rescue operation. However, if the NDRP is effectively implemented in respect of capacity building, it should be possible to improve on the lack of adequate human capacity.

Nigeria seems to have attempted a good start in bridging the capacity-building gap through two training programmes now available at the Master's level in the Institute of African Studies and Centre for Peace and Conflict Studies (CEPACS), both in University of Ibadan, and at the diploma level in LASU. There are also opportunities for collaboration in peace and conflict research in the country. For example, AREF has promoted one such centre in LASU while CEPACS collaborates with the Initiative on Conflict Resolution and Ethnicity (INCORE), University of Ulster, Derry/Londonderry, Northern Ireland in research and organization of conferences, seminars and workshops.

However, there is very little effort, if any at all in the area of short-term capacity building for government and NGO officials involved in conflict resolution and management and in particular, in health care delivery both under conflict and in post-conflict situations. This is another area that needs to be focused on urgently to ensure effective post-conflict health delivery in the West African subregion, perhaps, using as a springboard, the newly-founded institutions in Nigeria, and that is to develop partnerships and networks with other institutions in the subregion.

In spite of the existence of a Department of Relief and Rehabilitation in NEMA, its activities, as enunciated in the NDRP, are focused mainly on the short-term relief end. Besides, we found out that neither NEMA nor NCFR and in fact the FMOH, has any unit that coordinates the activities of NGOs, particularly NGOs to ensure that there are no duplication, wastages and redundancies in health care delivery both in conflict and in post-conflict situations. Also, our study did not reveal the existence of any guidelines or other instruments to do this. This will mean that the critical dilemmas of post conflict health care identified by Macrae (1997) may be difficult to contain in Nigeria. Accordingly, the study recommends the setting up of the appropriate unit to do this together with the necessary policy and guidelines to ensure that the dilemmas can be contained and sustainability of the health system under conflict assured.

Chapter Thirteen

THE ROLE OF ECOWAS AND OTHER REGIONAL HEALTH INSTITUTIONS IN POST-CONFLICT HEALTH CARE

13.1 Structure of ECOWAS in Relation to Health Care Delivery Under Conflict

When ECOWAS was established in 1975, its founding fathers envisaged it to become the single most important vehicle for economic cooperation and development in the West African subregion. However, since the late 1980s, the subregion seemed to have become a theatre of perennial intra-state conflicts. Given the potential impact of peace on health and correspondingly, that of health on development, one of the implicit visions of the founding fathers of ECOWAS is that it should be able to provide adequate health care under conflict situations including post-conflict health care. To be able to effectively accomplish this implies the existence of relevant institutional framework, human and material capacity for post-conflict health policy planning and health care delivery. In particular, Ajayi (2002) identified the lack of, or weaknesses of existing institutions, as constituting a major constraint to the growth and development process of Africa, in general, and Nigeria, in particular. Accordingly, the extent to which ECOWAS and its agencies are well prepared to meet the challenges of post-conflict health care, *ex ante*, should be of paramount importance to researchers and policy-makers. This is the focus of this section.

A major objective of ECOWAS is the harmonization and coordination of national policies and the promotion of integration programmes, projects and activities in about twenty sectors including health. Food, agriculture and natural resources, industry, transport and communications, trade, money and finance, are also areas and/or sectors of explicit focus, among others (Soyibo, 1999). In particular, Article 61 paragraph1(d) of the Revised ECOWAS Treaty, specifically enjoins Member States to 'encourage and strengthen cooperation among themselves in health matters'. As regards conflict resolution issues, addressed in Article 58(2) of the Revised Treaty, Member States are enjoined to 'cooperate with the Community in establishing and strengthening appropriate mechanisms for timely prevention of intrastate and interstate conflicts'. However, while protocols on Non-Aggression by Member States and on Mutual Assistance on Defence between Member States have been in existence for a long time, it was not until 10th December, 1999 that the protocol on the Mechanism for Conflict Prevention, Management, Resolution, Peace-Keeping and Security was ratified by Heads of State and Government of ECOWAS in Lome, Togo.

The West African Health Organization (WAHO) whose treaty was signed in Abuja, Nigeria on 9th July, 1987 is empowered by Article 2 of its protocol to takeoff through the merger of two subregional health organizations which were originally serving Anglophone and Francophone West Africa, respectively. The West African Health Community (WAHC) is the subregional health organization serving Anglophone West Africa while *Organisation de coordination et de Cooperation pour la Lutte contre les Grandes Endemies*(OCCGE) serves Francophone countries except the Republic of Guinea. WAHO is expected to serve all ECOWAS Member States, i.e. all five Anglophone countries, all ten Francophone countries and the two Lusaphone countries of Guinea-Bissau and Cape Verde.

The objective of WAHO 'shall be the attainment of the highest possible standard and protection of the health of the peoples in the subregion harmonization of the policies of Member States, pooling of resources, cooperation with one another and with others for a collective and strategic combat against the health problems of the subregion'[1] To achieve this objective, Article 3(2) of the Protocol prescribes fourteen odd functions for the organization, four of which can be creatively adapted to satisfy the requirements of health care delivery under conflict. These are to:

- assist in strengthening the health services and infrastructure of Member States where necessary;
- give active support to Member States in solving health problems in times of natural disasters or emergencies;
- collaborate with international, regional, and subregional organizations with a view to solving health problems in the subregion; and
- promote cooperation among scientific and professional groups which contribute to the advancement in health.[2]

Of the fourteen functions assigned to WAHO, only one can be seen to be explicitly linked to health care delivery under conflict. Even then, there does not seem to be any explicit concern for solving health problems arising from violent conflict except in as much as they only cause 'emergencies'. Thus, it appears that the only function assigned to WAHO in relation to health care delivery under conflict appears only concerned with providing relief, the short-term end of the relief-rehabilitation-development continuum of post-conflict health care. This appears to be a weakness in the framework of the West African subregion in relation to how it solves the problems arising from health care delivery under conflict.

In spite of this limitation in the design of WAHO, even this minimum specification in its protocol is yet to be implemented because of its inability to take off. Accordingly, while a lot seems to be known about ECOMOG, the military aspect of conflict management and resolution in the subregion, very few people, except perhaps health professionals and academics, know anything about WAHO, quite unlike the Pan-American Health Organization (PAHO), its counterpart in the Americas, which celebrated its centenary recently. It is also not as well known as its Eastern, Central and Southern African counterpart; the Commonwealth Regional Health Community Secretariat, based in Arusha, Tanzania and which in 2003, launched a resource mobilization drive for an Expanded and Comprehensive Response to the HIV/AIDS scourge in the subregion (Lambo, 2003).

There does not appear to be the political will from politicians of the subregion to break away from legacies of their colonial past epitomized by WAHO and OCCGE. This is also demonstrated in the approach adopted by Member States of ECOWAS in their objective of having a single currency. While the Francophone countries have one Central Bank, the BCEAO, and a single currency, the CFA franc, the Anglophones led by Nigeria and Ghana have decided to fast-track the establishment of a single currency, the Eco by 2005. Functionally, therefore, there are two major subregional health institutions in West Africa: WAHC and OCCGE.

The establishment of a Mechanism for Conflict Prevention, Management, Resolution, Peacekeeping and Security (MCPMRPS), by ECOWAS marked another milestone in the life of the Community. This formalized, in a more enduring fashion, the establishment of ECOMOG (ECOWAS Cease-fire Monitoring Group), and the subregional intervention force in the late 1980s to stem the tide of the ensuing civil war in Liberia. With the establishment of ECOMOG, many observers viewed the development as a departure from the Community's integration role (ECOWAS, 1999). However, given the negative impact which violence can have on the subregion's integration and economic development, it will be seen to in the right direction.

In addition to this development, sixteen Heads of State and Government of ECOWAS signed the, *Declaration of Moratorium on the Importation, Exportation and Manufacture of Light Weapons in West Africa* on 31st October, 1998. This Moratorium, commonly known as the West African Small

Arms Moratorium (WASAM), became effective on 1st November, 1998 for a renewable period of three years. It is an innovative approach for peace-building and conflict-prevention. Though, not a legally-binding regime, it is an expression of shared political will (Seck, 1999).

The MCPMRPS has a number of objectives specified in its protocol. Among these are:

- strengthen cooperation in the areas of conflict prevention, early-warning, peace-keeping operations, control of cross-border crime, international terrorism and proliferation of small arms and anti-personnel mines;
- maintain and consolidate peace, security and stability within the Community;
- establish institutions and formulate policies that would allow for the organization and coordination of humanitarian relief missions;
- promote cooperation between Member States in the areas of preventive diplomacy and peace-keeping;
- set up an appropriate framework for the rational and equitable management of natural resources shared by neighbouring Member States, which may cause frequent inter-state conflict; and
- formulate and implement policies on anti-corruption, money-laundering and illegal circulation of small arms.[3]

The mechanism carries out its functions and achieves its objectives through such institutions as *The Authority* composed of Heads of State and Government; the *Mediation and Security Council* made up of nine Member States: the Current Chairman and the immediate past Chairman and seven Member States elected by the Authority; and the *Executive Secretariat* headed by the Executive Secretary who shall have powers to initiate actions for conflict prevention, management, resolution, peace-keeping and security in the subregion.

There are three supporting organs of the institutions of the MCPMRPS:

- The *Defence and Security Commission* which shall meet once every quarter and shall examine all technical and administrative issues and assess logistical requirements for peace-keeping operations.

- The *Council of Elders* made up of eminent personalities identified by the Executive Secretary, on behalf of ECOWAS and who are expected to use their good offices and experience to perform the role of mediators, conciliators and facilitators.

- *ECOMOG*, a structure composed of several stand-by multi-purpose modules (civilian and military) in their country of origin and ready for immediate deployment. It is charged with eight missions:
  - Observation and Monitoring;

- Peace-keeping and restoration of peace;
- Humanitarian intervention in support of humanitarian disaster;
- Enforcement of sanctions including embargo;
- Preventive deployment;
- Peace-building, disarmament and demobilization;
- Policing activities including the control of fraud and organized crime; and
- Any other operations as may be mandated by the Mediation and Security Council.

The WASAM is being implemented through a tripartite collaborative arrangement involving the Programme for the Coordination and Assistance for Security and Development (PCASED) based in Bamako, Mali, and administered by the United Nations Development Programme (UNDP); the United Nations Regional Centre for Peace and Disarmament in Africa, based in Lome, Togo, and the ECOWAS Executive Secretariat in Abuja, Nigeria.

Among the activities defined by WASAM are the development of a culture of peace; training for security, military and police forces; enhancement of weapon controls at border posts; establishment of a database and a regional arms register; collection and destruction of surplus and unauthorized weapons; facilitation of dialogue with producers/ suppliers; review and harmonization of national legislation and administrative procedures; mobilization of resources for PCASED objectives and activities; and enlarging the membership of WASAM.

ECOWAS (1999) reported that the dialogue initiated soon after the declaration of WASAM led to an agreement with manufacturers and suppliers not to export arms to the subregion if the exporter had not been granted exemption. However, only five Member States have set up their National Commissions on the Control of Illicit Light Weapons Trafficking and Proliferation and most Member States have not forwarded their harmonized legislation on small arms control to the ECOWAS secretariat (ECOWAS, 2000a). This shows that even where there is some improvement in the development of the necessary framework at the regional level, the political will for the implementation at the national level appears lacking in most countries of the subregion.

13.2 Conflict Resolution and Management Experience in West Africa and Possible Post-Conflict Health Care Effects

Early in its existence, ECOWAS had been concerned with regional peace and security issues. Thus, in 1978, Heads of State and Government of the Community in 1978 adopted a non-aggression protocol, while a defence assistance protocol was adopted in 1981. In July 1991, the Heads of State and Government also adopted a declaration of political principles that asserts the primacy of democratic principles in the subregion and unequivocally condemned any seizure of political power force of arms. The Authority of Heads of State and Government of the Community also created the ECOMOG as a peace-keeping force following a series of violent conflicts in many West African countries. ECOMOG has had cause to intervene in Liberia, Sierra Leone and Guinea-Bissau and lately in Cote d'Ivoire.

ECOMOG was established mainly in response to the protracted civil war in Liberia. It was first deployed to the country in August 1990 where it worked to restore peace, ensure security, law and order. It also engaged in many humanitarian activities (including delivery) aimed at reducing the suffering of the people (ECOWAS, 2000b). However, the instrument establishing ECOMOG, explicitly gives its Commander power to 'arrange for necessary supporting units to provide medical, dental and sanitary services for all personnel..'[4], suggesting only officials of ECOMOG are explicitly to be catered *by* the group in terms of health care delivery. But this does not diminish the facilitation role of ECOMOG for health care delivery under conflict as a humanitarian operation. In fact, ECOWAS (2000b) asserted that ECOMOG, whose contingents were contributed by the eleven West African countries of Burkina Faso, Cote d'Ivoire, Gambia, Ghana, Guinea, Mali. Niger, Nigeria, Senegal, Sierra Leone and Togo, helped considerably in creating favourable conditions for the holding of free and fair elections in Liberia on 19th July 1997.

The intervention of ECOMOG forces in Sierra Leone came as a result of the overthrow of the democratically elected government of President Ahmed Teejan Kabbah. In February 1998, ECOMOG restored the lawful government of President Kabbah. The necessary measures taken to rekindle trust between warring parties by ECOMOG included the disarmament, demobilization and reintegration programme, which took off with the establishment of twenty-seven arm collection sites, ten demobilization centres and six arms storage centres (ECOWAS, 1999). A peace accord was negotiated between the restored government and all the antagonists in the conflict, namely the military junta, the Armed Forces Revolutionary Council (AFRC), the rebel Revolutionary United Front (RUF) and the government of President Kabbah in Lome, September 1999. This led to the return of the leaders of the AFRC, Lt. Col. Johnny Paul Koromah and

RUF, Corporal Fode Sankoh to Sierra Leone. This also led to the deployment of troops of the United Nations Observer Mission in Sierra Leone (UNOMSIL), following appeals made to the international community to give meaningful assistance to a final restoration for peace in the country.

The Executive Secretary of ECOWAS initiated the establishment of the MCPMRPS following the failure to resolve the crisis in Guinea-Bissau even after a number of cease-fire agreements were signed. Some units of the armed forces of Guinea-Bissau, led by the Chief of Defence Staff, rebelled against the government in June 1998. The President of the country requested for assistance from the Republic of Guinea and Senegal, two countries with which Guinea-Bissau had bilateral defence and security agreements. Based on the request of President J. B. Vieira, the Authority of Heads of State and Government of ECOWAS decided to restore peace and order and reinstated the democratically elected president. This it did and went further to establish a mechanism for supervision and control cease-fire manned by contingents from Benin, Niger and Togo. Yet, in spite of the numerous cease-fire agreements signed by the parties in conflict, the government was still overthrown (ECOWAS, 2000b).

This bitter experience led to the conception of the MCPMRPS in which emphasis is on conflict prevention rather than conflict resolution. The institutions and their supporting organs were discussed in the last section. In particular, the Executive Secretariat of the Mechanism is expected to establish an observation and monitoring system and a system of organs that would assist in containing and diffusing conflicts. The observation system will consist of a regional network of Member States grouped into zones. Four of such have been established with headquarters in Banjul, Gambia, and serving Cape Verde, Gambia, Guinea-Bissau, (Mauritania) and Senegal; Cotonou, Benin and serving Benin, Nigeria and Togo; Monrovia, Liberia and serving Ghana, Guinea, Liberia and Sierra Leone; and Ouagadougou serving Burkina Faso, Cote d'Ivoire, Mali and Niger.

The experience of conflict management and the resolution by ECOWAS in West Africa, though with a good beginning, lays a lot of emphasis on the military aspect, granted that the existence of peace is a *sine qua non* to other developments. Next is the consideration of relief and humanitarian activities. It is under this condition that health care delivery, both under conflict and post-conflict situations, falls. The health of survivors of conflict is very important and should be given the attention it deserves. The original ECOMOG regulations did not appear to give any explicit consideration to health care delivery beyond that involving its officials. This is a big limitation on ECOWAS legislation. Thus, the current conflict management and resolution experience of ECOWAS is likely to have very limited effects, if any at all, on health care delivery under conflict and in post-conflict situations.

Luckily, the protocol establishing the MCPMRPS recognizes ECOMOG as one of its three main institutions. Besides, it has broadened the structure of ECOMOG, conceiving it as consisting of stand-by multi-purpose civilian and military modules in Member States which can be called for deployment as and when needed. It has also broadened its roles and functions to include those that can be creatively exploited for effective health care delivery under conflict and post-conflict situations. These include the roles of:

- Humanitarian intervention in support of humanitarian disaster;
- Preventive deployment; and
- Any other operations as may be mandated by the Mediation and Security Council.

It is gratifying that this protocol recognizes explicitly the contributions of civilians to peace-keeping. This makes it easy for it to consider the problems of post-conflict health care delivery. It will be necessary, however to revise the ECOMOG regulations to take into cognizance this broadened outlook of ECOMOG as an agent of Conflict Prevention, Management, Resolution, Peace-keeping and Security. How well-equipped are the regional health institutions of ECOWAS in post-conflict health care delivery? We take up this issue in the next section.

13.3   Assessing the State of Readiness of ECOWAS Health Institutions For Health Care Delivery Under Conflict

We shall use the WAHC as a case study to evaluate the adequacy of the health institutions of ECOWAS for health care delivery under conflict and in post-conflict situations. WAHC came into existence on October 25, 1978 with the signing of its Treaty in Lagos by the Assembly of Health Ministers (AHM) of Member Countries, its highest policy organ.[5] The Community was established to undertake such activities as would contribute towards the attainment of the highest possible standards and protection of the health of the peoples of the Member Countries. It emphasizes the development and training of relevant human resources of all types and at all levels of the health care pyramid, particularly as it affects primary health care programmes. Among its objectives are:

- promoting activities designed to develop and strengthen Member Countries, public health services, health infrastructure and postgraduate medical and allied education; and
- facilitating cooperation between Member Countries and international health agencies in respect of health and social projects affecting Member Countries, and disseminating technical health information of interest (WAHC, 1999).

149

The functions of WAHC are carried out through its specialized agencies: the West African College of Surgeons and the West African College of Physicians; the West African Pharmaceutical Federation; and the West African College of Nursing. The major activities of the Community include:

- provision of Consultant Physicians, Surgeons and Peadiatricians, Pharmacists and Nurse Advisers, to serve in member countries;
- giving financial grants towards the training of medical personnel in institutions in Member Countries; and
- exchange of ideas and sharing of knowledge among health professionals and administrators of its Member Countries, through support for workshops, seminars, and update courses and research.

Clearly, the WAHC as presently constituted, appears inadequate to address issues relating to health care delivery under conflict and/or in post-conflict situations. However, it has features and characteristics like training, research and information dissemination infrastructures as specialized human capacity, that can be adopted and adapted for building the necessary institutional framework for health care delivery under conflict and in post-conflict situation.

Thus, ECOWAS and its agencies as presently constituted are not well equipped to deal with the problems and challenges posed by health care delivery under conflict. In recent times, particularly with the adoption of the MCPMRPS Protocol, there is a window of opportunity for adapting an existing framework to face these challenges. In the next section, we see how ECOWAS and its agencies can address the issues of health care delivery under conflict and in post-conflict situations in its Member States.

13.4 Future Roles for ECOWAS and Its Agencies for Health Care Delivery Under Conflict in West Africa

13.4.1 *Framework for Analysis*

For our analysis in this we adopt the framework proposed by Soyibo (1999). This framework takes into consideration five basic issues:

- the present framework of ECOWAS and its agencies in relation to health care delivery under conflict and post-conflict situations;
- impact of conflict on the health system;
- the Luxen (1997) principles for achieving the objectives of rehabilitation of the post-conflict health system;
- the three dilemmas confronting post-conflict health care rehabilitation (Macrae, 1997); and
- the basic principles of regional dimensions of conflict management and rehabilitation.

In this connection, we posit that for effective health care delivery under conflict and in post-conflict situations in the ECOWAS subregion, the roles to be played by the Community must be those that:

- build on the existing institutional infrastructure of ECOWAS, taking advantage of their potentials and reducing mutual suspicion between Member States;
- reduce to the minimum the negative impacts of conflicts on the health system;
- adapt the Luxen principle to the extent possible with a view to ensuring that an integrated and coordinated approach is employed for implementing the different phases of the relief-rehabilitation-development continuum;
- ensure that the dilemmas of legitimacy, sustainability and coherence that often confront the implementation of post-conflict health care programmes are reduced to the barest minimum; and
- enhance the positive values of regional approaches to conflict management and rehabilitation by diffusing potentials for hegemonic fears.

13.4.2 *The Proposition*

First, we propose that ECOWAS should adopt a holistic and coordinated approach to health care delivery in under- conflict and post-conflict situations in which post-conflict rehabilitation is done within the general framework of political-social-economic rehabilitation. This will ensure that the three dilemmas of legitimacy, sustainability and coherence are taken care of almost simultaneously. Political rehabilitation will ensure the legitimacy of the transitional government. A holistic approach will also ensure that all the dimensions of relief-rehabilitation-development continuum will be taken into consideration with a view to ensuring that the necessary caveat of bringing about sustainability is taken care of. Of course, cohesion will be assured because, right from the outset, the programme will be coordinated, ensuring that there is no duplication of efforts and the actions and action plans focus on the needs of the affected populations and systems, and that what is provided is not just what the donors want to give.

In this connection, until the adoption of the MCPMRPS Protocol, it can be said that the approach adopted by ECOWAS and its agencies for conflict management and peace promotion was *ad hoc* and reactive rather than being proactive. The approach is flawed from at least two perspectives. First, it is very restrictive, being only military in outlook and is concerned mainly with peace-keeping and later with peace-enforcement. Second, its implementation threw up hegemonic fears from Member States of the subregion which perceived Nigeria, rightly or wrongly, as having territorial

151

ambitions. The backlash of such fears is epitomized by the kidnapping of some members of the Nigerian contingent of ECOMOG in Sierra Leone.

The good news is that the MCPMRPS adopts this holistic approach which recognizes the importance of the political, social and economic dimensions of post-conflict health care delivery. Its three main institutions: *the Authority*; the *Mediation and Security Council*; and the *Executive Secretariat*, as well as their three organs: the *Defence and Security Commission*; the *Council of Elders* and *ECOMOG*, provide adequate institutional framework, which can be creatively employed, together with the proactive WAHO, if and when it decides to address the challenges posed by health delivery under conflict and post-conflict situations in West Africa.

However, ECOWAS will need to wake up from its stupor and implement the protocol of WAHO, but with an explicit mandate on the management of health care in under-conflict and post-conflict situations. WAHO and its component agencies will need to be strengthened organizationally and financially to be able to carry out this additional but important responsibility. It will need to go beyond 'routine' training of specialist health personnel to giving specialized training in health care provision in under-conflict and post-conflict situations. The colleges of WAHC and OCCGE can easily be adapted to do this critical assignment, perhaps with technical assistance from identified donor agencies and institutions, particularly using short-term training techniques. One of the identified problems of regional approaches to conflict management particularly in developing countries is lack of finance (DAC, 1997). Strengthening WAHO financially, particularly in relation to building capacity for health care delivery in under- conflict and in post-conflict situations may, therefore require that the financial contributions of Member States will need to be increased. Given that a lot of them are in arrears even in basic membership contributions as well as for services already rendered, nothing may be forthcoming from many Member States.[6] In this connection, financial assistance may need to be sought from outside the subregion.

An appropriate unit, charged explicitly with health care delivery in under- conflict and post-conflict situations will need to be created in WAHO. Currently, the WAHO protocol specifies four technical/specialized units for the organization:

- division of health manpower development;
- division of health research and disease control; ·
- division of technical assistance; and
- division of health management and information.[7]

It should be possible to create, within the division of technical assistance, a unit of Health Care Relief and Rehabilitation. This unit will be responsible for health care delivery in under- conflict and post-conflict situations. It will receive results of early warning of possible conflicts in the subregion from the Early Warning System of the

MCPMRPS. It will design and implement health policy in under-conflict and post-conflict situations in the subregion. In collaboration with the division of health research and disease control, the unit will study any ensuing conflict situation to identify the health needs and problems of the affected population and the health system. This will form the basis for the design of strategies and implementation framework referred to earlier. The unit will also liaise with other institutions and organs of the MCPMRPS, particularly ECOMOG with which it will work cooperatively in designing and implementing its health delivery programmes in under-conflict and post-conflict situations. This will ensure a holistic and well-coordinated programme design and implementation.

---

[1] Article 3(1) of the Protocol establishing the organization.
[2] Articles 3(2)(i, j, k, l) respectively of WAHO Protocol.
[3] Article 3 of the MCPMRPS Protocol.
[4] Section 27, ECOMOG Regulation, *Official Journal of ECOWAS*, Vol. 21, 1992, p.39.
[5] WAHC was first established as the Commonwealth West African Regional Health Secretariat in May 1972 by Governments of Gambia, Ghana, Nigeria and Sierra Leone. In May 1974, the Republic of Liberia was admitted and the word 'Commonwealth' was dropped from its name (WAHC, 1999).
[6] In the implementation of the ECOWAS monetary harmonization programme, for example, some countries are still not able to clear the arrears owed the West African Clearing House since 1985. The Clearing House became the West African Monetary Agency in 1993 with headquarters in Accra, Ghana (Soyibo, 1998).
[7] Article 10(1) of the WAHO Protocol.

PART FIVE

EPILOGUE

Chapter Fourteen

LOOKING AHEAD — IMPLICATIONS OF THE STUDY, RECOMMENDATIONS AND CONCLUSION

In this concluding chapter, we shall first give a summary of the findings of the study, and then discuss their implications as well as the limitations of the study before giving some suggestions on future areas of study in post-conflict health care delivery in the West African subregion. Finally, we shall express our view on what lies ahead in the future for health care delivery under-conflict and in post-conflict situations in West Africa and conclude with some remarks.

14.1 Summary of Findings

14.1.1 *The Socio-economic Profiles of Study Countries*

The conflict countries under study are generally poor. And conflict accentuated their poverty. For example, Guinea-Bissau's GDP contracted by 28.8% in 1998, the year the conflict began and when its effect was apparently most drastic. The Liberian[1] economy declined throughout the period under study, while that of Sierra Leone declined in three of the six years of study. Per capita gross national investment in the conflict countries was least in Sierra Leone where it varied between the least value of $130 in 1999 and 2000; and with the highest value of $200 in 1996. It was highest in Guinea-Bissau where it varied between the least value of $160 in 1998, the war year and the highest value of $230 in each of 1996 and 1997. Gross national savings as a percentage of GDP declined in 1998 and 2000 in Guinea-Bissau, and in all the years between 1995 and 2000, except 1999, in Sierra Leone. In particular, it declined by 14.3% in 2000. It is not surprising that all the governments of the conflict countries depended largely on deficit financing to fund government operation. This was as high as 12.7% of GDP in Guinea-Bissau in 1997; 10.4 % of GDP in 1998 in Sierra Leone; and 14.2% of GDP in 1985 in Liberia. It is also not surprising that the index of terms of trade declined throughout the period of study in Guinea-Bissau and Sierra Leone[2]. In spite of their poverty, debt service as a proportion of GDP in these countries is still significant. In Sierra Leone, for example, it was as high as 8.0% in 1995, 6.4% in 1996 and

157

5.9% in 2000. For Guinea-Bissau, it was 5.9% in 1995, 4.1% in 1996 and 4.0% in 1999. In Liberia, it was as high as 5.4% in 1984.

In contrast, the non-conflict countries are better off than the conflict countries in terms of GDP growth rate; even if there are some areas of relatively poor economic performance. In Cote d'Ivoire, for example, the growth rate of GDP was at least 5.8% between 1995 and 1998, but it declined sharply to 1.6% in 1999 and recorded a negative growth rate of 2.3% in 2000. Nigeria's performance is very much less impressive recording GDP growth rates of between 2.5% and 4.3% between 1995 and 1997. This dropped to 1.9% in 1998, rising to 3.8% in 2000. It is significant to note that Nigeria did not record any negative GDP growth rate during the period under study. Per capita gross national domestic investment is relatively impressive in Cote d'Ivoire. It is generally about three times the corresponding value of the other study countries. It was $650 in 1995, reaching the peak of $700 in 1997 before declining to $690 in 1998, $670 in 1999 and $660 in 2000. In contrast, Nigeria's per capita gross national investment was $210 in 1995, reaching the peak of $270 in 1997, before dropping to $260 in 1998, and $250 in 1999 and rising again to $260 in 2000. Gross national savings as percentage of GDP, is also relatively better in Cote d'Ivoire, although much lower than the stipulated threshold for industrial takeoff. It was 10.6% in 1995, rising to 12.4% in 1998, before declining to 11.9% and 9.6% in 1999 and 2000, respectively. Again, Nigeria's performance is not as good for most of the years, although, the performance in each of 1999 and 2000 seems to show some promise. It recorded 0.0% for the years 1995 – 1998, 13.9% in 1999 and 27.6% in 2000. The degree of deficit financing is not as pronounced in the non-conflict countries. In fact, it occurred only once in Nigeria during the period under study and that was in 1998 when it was 6.3% of GDP. In Cote d'Ivoire, its highest value was 4.1% in 1995, thereafter, it hovered around 2.2% and 2.9%. Cote d'Ivoire seems to have the highest debt burden among the study countries. This is exemplified by its relatively higher debt service as a percentage of GDP. It was 10.2% in 1995, rising to 12.3% in 1996, declining to 11.7% in 1997 and rising again to 12.4% in 1999. In Nigeria, debt service as a proportion of GDP was 6.3% in 1995, rising to 7.0% in 1996, falling to 4.0% and 2.5% in 1998 and 1999, respectively.

Health status in the conflict countries is, in general, low. Life expectancy in Guinea-Bissau for example is forty-four years in 1999. In Sierra Leone, it is thirty-seven years, and in Liberia it is fifty-two years, the African average. Infant mortality rate is 127 per 1000 in Guinea-Bissau; it is ninety-one in Liberia and 168 in Sierra Leone. The African average is eighty-seven per 1000. Maternal mortality rate is 910 per 100,000 live births in Guinea-Bissau; it is 560 in Liberia and 800 in Sierra Leone, compared to the African average of 734. The fertility rate is quite high in these countries. It is 5.8 per woman in Guinea-Bissau, 6.0 in Liberia and 5.9 in Sierra Leone, in contrast to the

African average of 5.2. Yet, health services and facilities are in short supply. In Guinea-Bissau, population per physician during 1990–1999 was 5,665 and 9,454 in Liberia. The proportion of the population that has access to safe water was 53% in Guinea-Bissau during 1990-98. It was 40% in Liberia and 34% in Sierra Leone, in comparison to the African average of 56%. Public sector expenditure in health care delivery is generally very low. It is estimated to be 1.1% of GDP in Guinea-Bissau and 1.0% in Sierra Leone, very much below the African average of 2.2%.

Health status is also poor in the non-conflict countries. Life expectancy was forty-six years in 1999 in both Cote d'Ivoire and Nigeria, well below the African average of fifty-four years. Infant mortality rate was 111 per 1000 live births in Cote d'Ivoire while in Nigeria; it was eighty-three, a little below the African average of eighty-seven. Maternal mortality rate in 1999, was 810 per 100,000 and in Nigeria, it was 1,000 while the African average was 734. Fertility rate is high also in the non-conflict countries. It was 4.9 in 2000, the African average in Cote d'Ivoire and 5.2 in Nigeria. Availability of health services in the non-conflict countries, though relatively better, still needs improvement. Population per physician during 1990-98, was 1,250 while in Nigeria, it was 5,208. The proportion of the population that has access to safe water was 65% in Cote d'Ivoire, higher than the African average of 56%. In Nigeria, it was 49%. Public sector expenditure in health is also abysmally low in the non-conflict countries, it is estimated to be 1.1% of GDP in Cote d'Ivoire in 1990-97 while in Nigeria, the corresponding value was 0.7%, well below the African average of 2.2%.

14.1.2 *Burden of Diseases*

Infectious diseases dominate the epidemiological pattern of the countries of study. Malaria has perhaps, the highest disease burden in these countries. In Guinea-Bissau, with diseases of the lower respiratory tract, diarrhea and tuberculosis, it accounts for about 38% of disease burden. It is estimated to cause about 20% to 30% of deaths in the country with a large burden of disease felt by older children and adults. In Liberia, it is estimated to attack about half of the population every year. It is one of the leading causes of death among under-fives, and of significant morbidity among other segments of the population. In Sierra Leone, the only malariometric survey conducted in 1977/79 showed that, malaria had a prevalence of 65.7% and is a leading cause of death among under-fives and of morbidity among other segments of the population. In Cote d'Ivoire, malaria and other infectious diseases like dysentery and pneumonia dominate the epidemiological environment. These diseases constantly put people off their daily activities, leading on average to a loss of 7.5 days and 7.9 days per month respectively for males and females in rural areas. In urban areas, they are estimated to cause a loss of 5.3 days per month. The Nigerian epidemiological environment is dominated by a high

159

prevalence of malaria infecting 919 per 100,000. This problem is aggravated by the existence of drug-resistant malaria whose occurrence is estimated to have increased from 2% in 1992 to 40% in 1996.

The spread of other diseases is causing concern to health authorities in the study countries. In Guinea-Bissau, the incidence of tuberculosis is of 361 per 100,000; higher than the sub-Saharan African average of 339 per 100,000. In Liberia, the overall prevalence of onchocerciasis is yet to be determined. This, with other infectious diseases like cholera, yellow fever and diarrhea, are a source of worry to the authorities. In Sierra Leone, the spread of onchocerciasis is a source of worry. It is estimated to have overall prevalence of 43% in the forest-savannah mosaic of the northern region and 85% of the forest zone of the south. In Cote d'Ivoire, dysentery is estimated to have a prevalence of 400 per 1,000 while pneumonia has a prevalence of 130 per 1,000. The epidemiological situation in the country is also characterized by other endemic diseases like dracunculiasis, schitosomiasis and onchocerciasis, which are sources of illness and are associated with a loss of productivity. Tuberculosis with a prevalence of 375 per 100,000 and other water borne diseases like diarrhea and typhoid are also becoming diseases of serious public health concern because of the poor quality of health infrastructure and obsolete equipment. In Nigeria, other diseases like dysentery with a prevalence of 386 per 100,000; pneumonia, 146 per 100,000 and measles, 89 per 100,000, are sources of increasing public health concern. Other endemic diseases like dracunculiasis, schistosomiasis, and onchocerciasis characterize Nigeria like Cote d'Ivoire, while the breakdown of public infrastructure has made the spread of water-borne diseases like diarrhea and typhoid, also a source of public health concern. Also, diseases like cerebrospinal meningitis, yellow fever and Lassa fever are occurring with increasing frequency in epidemic proportion.

14.1.3 *Assessment of the Impact of Conflict on the Health System*
The duration of conflict varied from one country to the other and affected health facilities differently. It lasted for about a year or so in Guinea-Bissau. It lasted much longer in Liberia and Sierra Leone. All the facilities surveyed in Guinea-Bissau indicated that the conflict lasted between 1998 and 1999. In Liberia, for most of the facilities surveyed (63.2%), the conflict began in 1989 while for 36.8% of the facilities, the conflict started in 1990. For most facilities (52.6%), the conflict lasted for eight years. For the remaining facilities, the conflict lasted for seven years. The conflict in Sierra Leone was more prolonged. For most facilities (92.3.9%), the conflict started in 1991 and lasted till the year 2000 for a majority (76.9%) of them. For 7.7% of the facilities surveyed the conflict lasted till 1999 and 2001. It was still on-going also in the case of 7.7% of the surveyed facilities at the time of our field visit. Thus, for a majority of the facilities (76.9%) surveyed in Sierra Leone, the conflict lasted for nine years.

One of the negative impacts of conflict on health facilities is that it often leads to a shut-down of operations. Our survey showed that in Guinea-Bissau, nearly 25% of the facilities that were surveyed were shut down during the conflict for a varying number of times. Of these, 17.9% were closed down only once while 3.6% were each closed down three and four times, respectively. In contrast, in Liberia, health facilities were shut down on an average of 1.71 times. Many facilities (42.1%) were shut down twice during the conflict while 21.2% were shut down only once. The proportion of surveyed facilities shut down three times was 14.8% while 5.3% of the facilities were shut down four times. On average, shutting of facilities as a result of conflict appeared to be more in Sierra Leone, perhaps due to its longer duration. On average, facilities were shut 1.78 times during the conflict. In particular, 22.2% of the facilities were shut down once, 48.1% twice, 14.8% three times and 3.7% four times during the conflict.

Conflict has negative effects on the human capital of the health system. Our study showed that in Guinea-Bissau, the conflict had differing impacts on the supply of the different personnel categories. Before the conflict, for example, there were, on average 2.30 doctors per facility. These dropped by 50.4% to 1.14 per facility during the first year of the conflict and marginally to 1.03 by 10% during the second year of the conflict. In Liberia, the average number of doctors per facility dropped by 15% from 9.41 before the conflict to 8.00 during the first year of the conflict. It dropped further by nearly 55% to 3.62 during the second year of the conflict. In Sierra Leone, a similar trend is observed, though on a smaller scale. The average number of doctors per facility dropped from 3.6 before the conflict by 27.8% to 2.6 during the first year of the conflict. In Guinea-Bissau, the effect of the conflict on the supply of nurses in the facilities was not as pronounced as that of doctors. Before the conflict, the average number of nurses per facility was estimated as 3.69 and this dropped by 4% to 3.55 during the first year of the conflict. It dropped further by 12.3% to 3.11 per facility during the second year of the conflict. In Liberia, the effect of the conflict on the supply of nurses was more drastic. The average number of nurses per facility dropped from 38.5 by more than 76% before the conflict to just 9.2 during the first year of the conflict. However, it remained virtually the same during the second year of the conflict. In Sierra Leone, the impact on the supply of nurses appeared to follow the pattern in Guinea-Bissau. The average number of nurses per facility dropped from 9.5 by 2.1% before the conflict to 9.3 during the first year of the conflict. The average number of pharmacists per facility in Guinea-Bissau dropped from 2.18 by 31.2% before the conflict to 1.50 per facility during the first year of the conflict. It dropped further by 22% to 1.17 during the second year of the conflict. In general, in Liberia, there appears to be a general shortfall in the supply of pharmacists in the health facilities. Thus, the average number of pharmacist per facility which was 0.75

before the conflict dropped by 4% to 0.72 during the first year of the conflict and dropped further by 1.4% to 0.71 during the second year of the conflict. In Sierra Leone, the average number of pharmacists per facility was increased by 16.6% from 1.8 before the conflict to 2.1 during the first year of the conflict. This may be the result of substitution of skill categories as a result of conflict.

The supply of health personnel tended to improve with the cessation of hostilities. The average number of doctors per facility in Guinea-Bissau increased by 48.6% from 1.40 during the first year after the conflict to 2.08 in the second year after the conflict. In Liberia, the increase in the average number of doctors after the conflict increased marginally by nearly 5 % between the first and second years after the conflict. In Sierra Leone, the average number of doctors increased by 54% from 2.4 and 3.7 between the first and second years after the conflict. Among nurses, peace has a much more salubrious effect on the supply in most study countries. In Liberia, the average number of nurses per facility increased by over 120% from 9.11 to 20.1 between the first year after the conflict and the second year after the conflict. Similarly, the supply of nurses after the conflict in Sierra Leone increased by 124% from 9.3 to 20.9 between the first year after the conflict and the second year after the conflict. However, in Guinea-Bissau, the supply of nurses experienced a slight decline of about 2% between the first year after the conflict and the second year after the conflict. The supply of pharmacists improved in Guinea-Bissau under the post-conflict situations by 28.7%. In Liberia, where facilities tended to suffer from the lack of pharmacists, the effect of relative peace was more dramatic, improving supply by over 108%, from an average of 0.68 per facility to 1.42 between the first and second years after the conflict.

Conflict also leads to the destruction of health infrastructure. The number of functioning wards in Guinea-Bissau declined by 23.7% from an average of 8.87 per facility to 6.77 during the first year of the conflict. This further declined by 16.7% to 4.64 in the second year of the conflict. In Liberia, the average number of functioning wards dropped from 4.87 per facility to 3.77, a decrease of 21.0% during the first year of the conflict. In Sierra Leone the number of functioning wards decreased by 6.5% from an average of 6.2 per facility to 5.8 during the first year of the conflict. It decreased marginally further by 2% during the second year of the conflict. With peace, there is some improvement in the availability of infrastructure, although rehabilitation of infrastructure is more of a long-term solution of the post-conflict health system. In spite of this, in Guinea-Bissau, the average number of functioning wards increased dramatically from 5.64 per facility to 11.67, an increase of 106.9%, between the second year of the conflict and the first year after the conflict. This was further increased marginally by 14.1% to 12.54 between the first and second years after the conflict. In Liberia, post-conflict situations brought an improvement in the availability of functioning wards. The number of functioning wards increased from an average of 4.36 per facility during the first year after the conflict by 24% to 5.42 during the second year after the conflict. In Sierra Leone, the average number of functioning wards increased from 5.7 to 6.4 by 12% between the cessation of hostilities and the second year after the conflict.

Conflict also has effects on service delivery at the facility level. The literature of health care delivery under conflict suggests that health resources tend to be diverted to treat more pressing war-related health conditions. This may lead in some cases to an increase in patients in facilities that are not shut down due to the conflict. It may also lead to a fall in the number of patients, due to inaccessibility problems posed by the conflict. In Guinea-Bissau, the average number of outpatients increased by 77.3% during, the first year of the conflict. During the second year of the conflict, the average number of outpatients per facility increased by nearly 107.7%. In Liberia, the average number of out-patients per facility before the conflict was 34,790. This fell by 35.8% to 22,330 during the first year of the conflict. It fell further by 4% to 22,330 during the second year of the conflict. Similarly, the average number of in-patients fell from 1,768 before conflict by 23.4% to 1,354 during the first year of the conflict. It fell marginally further by 2.4% to 1,322 during the second year of the conflict. In Sierra Leone, there was an increase of 23% in the average number of out-patients per facility during the first year of the conflict. However, there was an overwhelming increase in the average number of in-patients by 437% from 205.8 before the conflict to 1,106.8 during the first year of the conflict. With the cessation of hostilities there was a fall in the average number of out-patients and in-patients. The number of outpatients fell by nearly 18% from 1,347.9 to 1,107.2 during the second year after the conflict. The number of in-patients fell by 28% from 919.3 a year after the conflict to 616.7 two years after the conflict.

Conflict has deleterious effects on the health management process too. In Guinea-Bissau, the facilities that were surveyed reported having 1.58 management meetings on average per facility before the conflict. This dropped by 63.3% to 0.58 during the first year of the conflict. And further, by nearly 97% to 0.02 during the second year of the conflict. In Liberia, surprisingly, there was a marginal increase in the average number of management meetings held per facility by 2.2% from 9.20 to 9.40 before the conflict and the first year of the conflict. However, with the onset of the conflict, a significant reduction in the number of management meetings was experienced. Thus, the average number of management meetings held per facility fell from 9.40 during the first year of the conflict by about 29% to 6.70 during the second year of the conflict. In Sierra Leone, the frequency of management meetings held per facility decreased from an average of 6.6 per facility before the conflict by about 29% to 4.7 during the first year of the conflict.

Another negative effect of conflict on the management process of health facility is the limitation on the maintenance function of the facilities' human capital. An index for measuring this is the decrease in the average number staff exposed to training. In Guinea-Bissau, the conflict seemed to affect the exposure of health facility staff to training. Before the conflict, on average, 14.33 staff per facility was exposed to training. During the first year of the conflict, this dropped sharply by several multiples to 0.01 per facility. In fact, during the second year of the conflict, none of the staff of the facilities that were surveyed attended any training. In general, personnel of the health facilities surveyed in Liberia tended not to be exposed to training, as a matter of practice. Thus, on average, less than one personnel per facility indicated attending training per year. In spite of this, the conflict still had its negative effect, however, marginal. Before the conflict and during the first year of the conflict, the average number of staff that attended training fell from 0.38 per facility by 5.3% to 0.36. But between the first year of the conflict and the second year, the decrease in the proportion of staff exposed to training per facility widened by more than three-fold to 16.7%! In the case of Sierra Leone, the average number of staff exposed to training per facility fell from 3.0 before the conflict to 2.6 during the first year of the conflict, a decrease of 13%.

Cessation of hostilities is expected to bring about improvement in the number of staff exposed to training. In Guinea-Bissau, from a nil number of staff sent for training during the second year of the conflict, the average number of staff sent for training per facility rose to 3.8 per facility during the first year after the conflict. However, this dropped by nearly 98% to 1.00 during the second year of the conflict. In Liberia, under post-conflict situations, the average number of staff sent for training improved by more than four-fold, from a value of 0.32 per facility during the first year of the conflict to 1.73 during the second year of the conflict. In Sierra Leone, the expected increase in the number of staff attending training under post-conflict situations did not materialize. Rather, the average number of staff attending fell from 2.4 per facility a year after the conflict by 29% to 1.7 two years after the conflict. The possible reasons for this type of unexpected result may be the lack of funds for training or non-availability of the specific type of training required for a more overwhelming number of staff. It may also be due to fear created in staff by the activities of RUF in many areas of the country.

14.1.4 *The Role of NGOs under Conflict*

NGOs are known to play important roles in health care delivery under conflict. Many of the NGOs appeared to be in operation mainly in response to the problems posed by the recent conflict in the study countries. Of the three NGOs surveyed in Guinea-Bissau, one began operation in 1996 while the remaining two began operation in1997. Returns from seven of the fifteen NGOs that were surveyed in Liberia were found usable and all of them were NNGOs. Their operations also appeared to be in response to the conflict as only one (14.1%) was in operation before the conflict. In the case of Sierra Leone, where twenty NGOs were surveyed with seventeen usable questionnaires retrieved, 70.6% of the NGOs were domestic and 41.2% started operation in the country after the commencement of hostilities. In Guinea-Bissau, the average number of health staff per NGO increased from nineteen during the first year of the conflict by 42.1% to twenty-seven during the second year of the conflict. Though, it declined to twenty during the first year after the conflict, it increased by 50% to 30 during the second year after the conflict. In Liberia, hostilities appeared to restrict the functioning of NGO staff as the average number of staff per NGO from thirty-six during the first year of conflict by 6% to thirty-four during the second year of the conflict. The average number of staff per NGO in Sierra Leone fell from 27.3 during the first year of the conflict by 8.0% to 24.9 during the second year of the conflict. During the first year after the conflict, the average number of health staff per NGO increased by 41% to 35.2.

In Guinea-Bissau, the average number of doctors per NGO surveyed was one before the conflict, this increased to two during the first year of the conflict and five during the first year after the conflict. The average number of nurses per NGO in Guinea-Bissau was ten during the first and second years of the conflict. It dropped to 5.5 in the first year after the conflict when there was a dramatic increase in the number of doctors per NGO. It would appear there was a substitution of doctors for nurses during the year by the NGOs surveyed. In the case of Liberia, the average number of doctors per NGO fell from 3.80 by nearly 16% to during the first year of the conflict to 3.20 during the second year of the conflict. The average number of nurses fell to about 7% from 17.40 to 16.30. In the case of Sierra Leone, the average number of doctors per NGO declined from 5.4 to 5.2 between the first and second years of the conflict, rising to 8.4 by about 62% during the first year after the conflict. This is also 64% of the average number of doctors during the second year after the conflict. This general statement can be made about all other NGO personnel categories in our sample, in the country.

It was difficult to make a general statement about the pattern of spending for health care delivery by NGOs surveyed. This was due to a number of reasons. First, the lack of financial data in some of the countries and the differing sample sizes. In Guinea-Bissau, for example, we did not obtain useful financial information from any of the three NGOs that returned completed questionnaires. Accordingly, we can only make conjectures about NGO health spending in this country using other facts available to us. Our survey of government officials, for example, indicated that interventions from NGOs and donor agencies like UNICEF, WHO and *Catholica Nationale* helped in reducing costs of health care during the crisis. We also found that in the facilities surveyed, the average actual expenditure tended to exceed the budget. For example, during the first year of conflict, the budget per facility dropped by 50% while actual expenditure increased by the same proportion. Besides, during the same period, the average actual expenditure/budget ratio per facility was 103%. We conjectured that the contributions of development partners and other stakeholders like NGOs, particularly NNGOs, must have boosted the spending of health facilities to attain this level. In the case of Liberia, our data indicated that the average amount spent on health by the NGOs in our sample, tended to decrease with increasing years of hostilities. This fell marginally by 3% during the second year of conflict to L$3.70 million. In the case of Sierra Leone, NGOs appear to spend more on average than the health facilities surveyed; though only a few of the NGOs supplied financial information. During the second year of conflict, for example, the average amount spent on NGO operations per organization was 6.3 million Leones, the minimum being 7.4 million Leones and the maximum, 15.1 million Leones. During the first year after the conflict, the average NGO expenditure per organization increased to 31.8 million Leones, which is four times more than the average amount spent during the second year of the conflict. The maximum was 108 million Leones while the minimum was 12 million Leones. This suggests that NGOs appear to contribute a lot to post-conflict health care in terms of the provision of funds.

14.1.5 *The Role of Government Under Conflict*
The role of government in health care delivery is affected by the level of institutional and policy framework in existence in the country of study. In general, the Ministry of Health is the main government agency in charge of health care delivery both in peacetime and under conflict. All the countries have at least one health plan or policy under which the health system operates. Guinea-Bissau appears to be the least developed and sophisticated in terms of the operations of the health system both in peacetime and under conflict. The health system still operates the 1976 Health Plan, which emphasizes decentralization of services, preventive care and the use of simple techniques and practices as well as training of all personnel types including volunteer staff like village health workers. Our survey shows that the Ministry of Public Health (MINSAP) which oversees health provision at all levels of governance in the country has no formal policy for health care delivery under conflict. It relies heavily on the 1976 Plan and on interventions from international agencies like UNICEF, UNDP and WHO, for implementing its health care delivery programmes.

In terms of personnel, the country suffers from a dearth of qualified personnel, particularly with the effects of the civil war. Many of the health centres are without nurses, not to talk of doctors. The village health posts (USBs) are based on community-participation with a significant amount of local-resource mobilization and sharing of responsibility between community leaders/members in the villages and MINSAP defined by contract letters between the relevant parties. However, the effective performance of the system is highly constrained by the high level of poverty of the citizenry in spite of their high level of enthusiasm. The high shortage of skilled manpower in the country's health system is also, in part, a reflection of the absence of tertiary and other professional institutions like a university for building such high human capital capacity in the country. Thus, it can easily be seen that it will be more difficult to get specialized training relating to health care delivery under conflict and in post-conflict situations in the country.

In Liberia, our survey reveals that the Ministry of Health and Social Welfare (MHSW) is the only government agency responsible for health care delivery under conflict situations in the country. But intra-sectoral collaboration of health care issues at the national level is promoted through an *ad hoc* committee, the Technical Advisory Committee (TAC) and the Health Services Coordinating Committee (HSCC). The TAC includes senior representatives of the MHSW, the WHO, UNICEF and other development partners. Representation on the HSCC includes all members of the fourteen County Health Teams (CHTs) and NGOs participating in the health sector. At the county operational level, the CHTs conduct meetings aimed at improving health services provision, developing joint plans of action, and agreeing on solutions to problematic programme areas. Our survey revealed that the relationship between the MHSW and members of the HSCC has been cordial and that NGOs are perceived as contributing immensely to national development.

The role of the GOL in meeting the challenges of post-conflict health care delivery is constrained by the availability of funds. For example, the post-war health budgets of the GOL were much lower than the pre-war budgets. Public allocation to health in 1981 was 10.2% of the total budget. However, in 1990, during the war, it was 5.6% of a smaller national budget. During the war, the only veritable spending on health by the public sector was on payment of salaries.

To meet the financing gap, the GOL had always sought refuge in emergency and humanitarian assistance provided by the country's growing and vibrant NGO sub-sector. For example, the spending of overseas development assistance in the health sector was characterized as 'robust in comparison to public sector spending'. Thus, in 1998, donors financed the major share of spending in the health sector in the country estimated to be US$25.4 million. However, donor releases tended to be lower than allocations. In 1997, for example, when Liberia was allocated US$100.7million ODA, the disbursements were actually 23.7% lower than 1996 while disbursements since 1996 averaged 20% of pledges. Worse still, it is expected that such assistance would continue to fall, given changes in the country's assistance status and other considerations.

The health system of Liberia is operated under the aegis of the National Health Policy (NHP) which seeks to: prioritize PHC services; transfer responsibility to lower health management levels; empower people to be more involved in their health care; nurture and strengthen partnerships for health development; mobilize local and external resources in support of health; and generate the political will to provide resources required for effective implementation of health and social welfare programmes

In Sierra Leone, the Ministry of Health and Sanitation is the only government agency involved in health care delivery under conflict or emergency situations. However, there is a unit of the Ministry which coordinates the activities of NGOs. Among such NGOs are the Sierra Leone Red Cross Society, Save the Children of Sierra Leone, Caritas Makeni, Care International; Leones and Cents and Planned Parenthood Association of Sierra Leone. Even before the beginning of hostilities, the health care delivery system of Sierra Leone had reached an appalling state of deterioration in quality and scope. Not a single Government Hospital was effectively functional. For example, Connaught Hospital, the biggest referral hospital in the country presented the sight of a severely overused institution with structures and facilities completely decayed or in a severe state of disrepair.

Under this appalling situation, the role of the Government of Republic of Sierra Leone (GOROS), was to lead the way in the rehabilitation of the wards of the different hospitals supported by individuals and business houses within the country. Funds were also obtained from Development Finance Institutions like the African Development Bank (ADB) and the World Bank. In terms of improvement in drug supplies the World Health Organization (WHO) and the United Nations Children's Fund (UNICEF) supported funding the cost recovery programme of government.

A number of policy guidelines and instruments were used to guide the operations of the Sierra Leonean health system. The first is the NHP, first developed in 1993 with specific goals for different areas of health care delivery and management like administration; financing; manpower development; infrastructure and transportation; primary health care; secondary and tertiary health care; private practice; drugs and medical supplies; control of communicable diseases; nutrition; information system and education; and legal aspects of health, among others. The second is the NHAP which built on the NHP and was developed in 1994. It outlines the main steps needed to develop a more effective, efficient and equitable health system. It gave decentralization of the health system top priority. This will involve creation of new leadership teams at lower levels, like the district level to be headed by district medical officers (public health) or district medical officers (clinical). At this level, the NHAP seeks to give additional training in the skills of the Community Health Officers to staff at the district level without primary health skills. As part of the decentralization process, the NHAP proposed the provision of a basic range of facilities at the village level and a wider range at health centres located in chiefdom headquarters and small towns. This document also seeks to promote cooperation and dialogue between government and NGOs with a view to translating the latter's useful and welcome support in a more positive and operationally more transparent perspective.

Our study showed that the breakdown of law and order as a result of the conflict led to the inability to operate the management framework proposed by the NHP and NHAP as part of the policy reforms of the health sector in the country. It also revealed that closure of facilities is perhaps, the most important impact of conflict in health care delivery in the country. With it, there would be fewer facilities to coordinate and monitor, if any. Where there were facilities operating, emphasis was shifted to curative care to the detriment of all aspects of health care like preventive care and public health, in general. Government was therefore unable to fulfill its expected role in health provision. Besides, as there is no specific agency of government charged with post-conflict health care *ab initio*, it certainly was an uphill task for government to overcome problems posed by conflict and its aftermath on the health system.

14.1.6   *The Potentials for Post-Conflict Health Care   in Cote d'Ivoire*
In Côte d'Ivoire, there are policies and procedures for the delivery of health care in emergency situations. However, there are no special policies and procedures for the delivery of health care in post conflict/emergency situations. The instruments, policies and guidelines (including laws) available to deliver health care during emergency and post conflict situations are the 'red plan' ('plan rouge') and 'ORSEC plan' ('plan ORSEC'). The objective of the Red Plan is to mitigate the consequences of an accidental or emergency situation, taking into account the following imperatives: the urgency of the putting into place of the means of intervention; the rational implementation of the plan; the use of sufficient and appropriate means; and the co-ordination of the implementation of the means of medical intervention.

There are two government agencies designated to provide emergency health care during conflicts or other forms of emergency. These are (a) the *Service d'Aide Médicale d'Urgence* (SAMU), that is Emergency Medical Help Service and hence providing only medical services; and (b) The fire brigade, called *Groupement des Sapeurs Pompiers Militaires* (GSPM), a branch of the armed forces, which provides assistance during fire outbreaks, health emergencies and accidents.

During emergency situations, an advanced medical post is created outside the disaster area to administer first aid health care services. The intervention group is made up of doctors, nurses, the fire brigade and first aid workers. This group is charged with the responsibility of collecting the victims and taking them to a more advanced medical post, where they will be prepared for evacuation. At the more advanced medical post, a first diagnosis is made to ascertain whether an ambulance or helicopter can evacuate them (major public or private hospitals, and clinics). Before that, the Medical Director of SAMU must collect information from all the hospitals to determine the number of persons they can receive.

The government of Cote d'Ivoire is the major source of funding these two agencies, although supplementary funding is obtained through external assistance particularly from the European Union (European Development Fund), and the World Health Organization (WHO), among others.

Our fieldwork revealed that the two agencies require more material, human and financial resources to carry out their work effectively. In the area of material resources, they need more cars, ambulances, helicopters, technical materials, and medical consumables. In particular, the GSPM indicated that it needed at least six medical doctors and drivers. In addition, all the materials the organizations currently have are old while their equipment needs replacement. They also need money to replace or repair some of the equipment that have broken down.

To solve these problems, the agencies proposed that the government increases their financial allocation in order that they can meet their requirements. The fire brigade (GSPM) indicated that in the last couple of years, it had been expecting to get additional allocation from government to pay its accumulated expenditures. In the same way, the government has to increase its human resources. To receive external assistance, the agencies would prefer direct assistance with government monitoring how the monies are spent. In particular, the fire brigade would prefer to repair all its grounded equipment by creating its own internal maintenance unit. In addition, with respect to external agencies, the two local agencies propose that the Health Minister signs a memorandum of understanding with such external bodies, on their behalf to enable them get more financial assistance to meet the demands of any ensuing emergencies.

These two agencies complement one another. Thus, they work together in emergency situations. In normal times, the SAMU, in order to handle emergencies, hires army medical officers from GSPM and pays them. With regard to emergency situations, particularly, it is the Prefect who coordinates all the activities requiring emergency assistance or help. However, there are no formal relationships between the two government agencies and the NGOs specializing in the health care delivery under emergency situations. When the services of NGOs are required, SAMU or the Prefect gets in contact with them and enters an operational contract for mitigating the situation. The NGOs are mainly 'Croix Rouge' (Red Cross) of Côte d'Ivoire, 'SOS Médecins' and 'Allo Docteurs', and 'l'Ordre de Malte', which offer drugs for those admitted to hospitals/clinics.

The International Federation of Red Cross and Red Crescent Societies (IFRC) is one of the major NGOs operations in the country and the West African subregion to mitigate the problems of health care delivery under conflict. Its mission in West Africa is to support and encourage the West African National Red Cross and Red Crescent Societies in sixteen countries, including Côte d'Ivoire, in meeting the needs of their most vulnerable residents. Apart from carrying out relief operations to assist

170

victims of disasters and strengthening of its member National Societies, it focuses on promoting humanitarian values, disaster response, disaster preparedness, and health and community care. With regard to health care, the focus is on: improved preparation and response to epidemics; reinforced awareness and prevention of HIV/AIDS; support and coordination of West African national societies' community based first aid (CBFA) projects; support to West African national societies' basic health care services; and reduced incidence of female genital mutilation.

14.1. 7 *The Potentials for Post-Conflict Health Care in Nigeria*

A number of attempts have been made to mortify post-conflict/emergency situations in Nigeria since the attainment of independence in 1960. The first major attempt was the establishment of the Nigerian Red Cross Society (NRCS) through an Act of Parliament in 1960, and its incorporation in 1961. In addition, some government parastatals/departments like the Nigeria Police Force, Nigeria Armed Forces, The Nigeria Fire Service, and some Non-Government Organizations (NGOs), are all stakeholders in conflict/emergency management in the country.

However, due to the inadequacies of existing government agencies to handle the emergency situations at the end of the Nigerian civil war (1967-1970), came the need to establish an appropriate institutional framework to take care of the needs of several hundreds of thousands of war victims. Accordingly, Decree 48 of 1976 was promulgated to establish an agency with the mandate of providing relief for, and engage in the rehabilitation of civil war victims. On board came the new agency, known as the National Emergency Relief Agency (NERA) which was, as its name suggests, basically relief-oriented. But, soon NERA became incapable of handling these situations because of several factors such as limited instruments, policy guidelines, and inadequate human and capital resources, among others.

Subsequently, the National Emergency Management Agency (NEMA), as a metamorphosis of NERA, was established through Decree 12 on 23 March 1999. Its establishment marked the first major attempt at comprehensively addressing problems arising from conflict and emergency situations in Nigeria. Over time, a number of policy guidelines and instruments for the operations of NEMA have been developed. If these are fully implemented, it should be possible to address many of the pressing issues thrown up by many of the conflict/emergency situations plaguing the country.

NEMA is saddled with the responsibility of coordinating the activities of all disaster management bodies such as, the International Red Cross and Red Crescent Society (IRCS), Nigeria Red Cross and Red Crescent Society (NRCS), local NGOs and CBOs, the organized private sector (construction consortiums like Julius Berger, big oil companies like Chevron Oil or Shell Petroleum Development Company etc), Military and Paramilitary agencies, etc. The decree establishing NEMA also made provision for each state of the Federation to set up a State Emergency Management Committee with spelt-out functions which include; notification of the apex agency (NEMA) of any natural or other disasters occurring within the state, responding to disasters and seeking for assistance from NEMA where necessary, etc.

NEMA's department of Relief and Rehabilitation attends to the basic needs of disaster/conflict victims in terms of the provision of food, shelter, water, medical care and the restoration of essential public utilities. It works in close collaboration with the NRCS which has a longer standing coverage in this field (the total number of volunteers of the IRCS as at 2001 is estimated at 105 million worldwide). The NRCS has a total of 250,000 volunteers in Nigeria alone. In addition, it also works in close collaboration with other NGOs in disaster management. The relief and rehabilitation work of the agency is not limited to the shores of Nigeria alone; but extends to other African nations like Chad, Niger, Liberia, etc.

Apart from its main function of formulating policies and guidelines and providing support to lower tiers of government, the Federal Ministry of Health (FMOH), also heads a National Committee on Emergency Preparedness and Response which the Honourable Minister of Health chairs. The National Committee on Emergency Preparedness and Response has a membership, which is drawn from international bodies like the World Health Organization (WHO), United Nations Children's Fund UNICEF); NGOs like the Red Cross and Red Crescent Society etc.

Besides, all Nigeria's General and Specialist Hospitals are responsible for the management of health cases arising from conflicts and emergencies. They are to manage the cases with a view to ameliorating the suffering of the victims and to control outbreaks of disease affecting victims or that might result from the conflicts/disasters. These institutions are responsible for health care management without discrimination in conflict and emergency situations especially those resulting from fire, accident and bomb or oil pipe-line blasts to ensure that lives of victims are saved.

Apart from international NGOs, a few indigenous NGOs exist in the area of conflict/emergency management in Nigeria. Perhaps, foremost amongst them is the African Refugee Foundation (AREF) which was established in 1994 by Ambassador Segun Olusola in response to the overwhelming demands of the Rwandan genocide by the majority Hutu population of the minority Tutsi ethnic group or their Hutu sympathizers. It has been involved in complex emergencies and disasters in many African countries like Ethiopia, Eritrea, Burundi, etc. In collaboration with *Doctors for all Nations*, it was involved in health care delivery under conflict in the horn of Africa by providing non-prescription medicines and other supplies. AREF has its own corps of medical and health volunteers who can be mobilized and allocated to areas of conflict at very short notice. In spite of this promise, AREF stills has limitations in the area of health care delivery under conflict,

172

and it needs more formal and careful planning in this regard. It has also collaborated with Lagos State University (LASU) to establish a research centre in peace and conflict studies and to build capacity for conflict resolution and management through a diploma course in peace and conflict studies. However, this does not contain formal training in health care delivery under conflict/emergency situations.

NEMA has developed an operations-oriented document, the National Disaster Response Plan (NDRP) that describes the mechanism by which the Federal Government mobilizes resources and conducts activities aimed at addressing the consequences of any major disaster or emergency that overwhelms the capacity of state and local governments in the country. To carry out the activities specified in the NDRP, NEMA, through signed letters of agreement, cooperates with a number of Federal Ministries, departments and agencies. The signatories to this agreement are the Federal Ministry of Aviation, the Federal Ministry of Health, the Federal Ministry of Transport, the Federal Ministry of Works and Housing, Ministry of Agriculture, Ministry of Power and Steel, Ministry of Foreign Affairs, Ministry of Internal Affairs, Ministry of Water Resources, Ministry of Finance, Ministry of Environment, Nigerian National Petroleum Corporation, National Electric Power Authority, Defence Headquarters, Nigeria Police, Nigerian Red Cross Society and NEMA. The NDRP is made of three parts:

- The basic plan which presents the policies and concepts of operations that guide how the Federal Government will assist disaster-stricken states and local governments. It also summarizes federal planning assumptions, response and recovery actions.
- Support Services Areas section which describes the mission, policies, concept of operations, and responsibilities of the primary and support agencies involved in the implementation of the key response functions that supplement state and local activities. SSAs include Transport, Communications, Public Works and Engineering, Firefighting, Information and Planning, Mass Care, Resource Support, Health and Medical Services, Search and Rescue, Hazardous Materials, Food, Energy and Military/Police Support.
- The Recovery Function section describes the policies, planning considerations, and concept of operations that guide the provision of assistance to help disaster victims and the affected communities return to normal life and minimize the risk of future damage. Assistance given is categorized by delivery system -either to individuals, families, and businesses or to states and local governments.

The NDRP is a comprehensive document. It contains important information, including addresses and telephone numbers about the agencies and officials to contact

173

in the event of any disaster. Among such agencies and/or officials are NEMA (with emergency hot lines specified); the three arms of the armed forces; in particular, the Nigerian Army and the Nigerian Air Force Disaster Response Units; the Federal Road Safety Corps; the Federal and State Fire Services; the Officials of the FMOH to contact in the event of any epidemic outbreak; the state command of the Nigeria Security and Civil Defence Corps; and the list of government hospitals, by state.

Thus, given the way the NDRP is designed and formulated, it has the potential for being adapted for health care delivery under conflict and in post-conflict situations. It is quite comprehensive and integrated, with health care being just a part of the disaster management. However, it focuses mainly on the short-term end of the relief-rehabilitation-development continuum.

The National Commission for Refugees (NCFR) is another agency of government responsible for conflict/emergency management in Nigeria. Established under Decree 59 of 1989 (Cap 244 Law of the Federation of Nigeria, 1990), it is the main instrument for the protection and management of refugees in Nigeria. The NCFR is concerned with refugees who are victims of war and other internal conflicts particularly in the West African subregion. As a result of the perennial crisis in the subregion, in the last decade or so, national refugee camps were set up in Oru, Ogun State and Maiduguri, Borno State. The management of the camp inmates is a collaborative work between the NCFR, NGOs and international donor agencies such as Caritas, UNICEF and the IRCS, etc. With the dramatic increase in communal violence in Nigeria, since the return of civilian rule in 1999, nearly all parts of the country have been plunged into a number of conflicts which are classified mainly as indigene-settler conflicts; inter-ethnic or intra-ethnic conflicts; intra or inter political parties conflicts, religious conflicts This has increased the phenomenon of internally displaced persons (IDPs) in Nigeria to well above 750,000 in 2003. Accordingly, the original mandate of the commission, which concerns mainly the welfare of refugees, was expanded to incorporate the welfare of IDPs. Thus, the NCFR focuses on the medium to a long-term end of the relief-rehabilitation-development continuum. However, there is no formal recognition for the role of the organization in health care delivery under conflict or in post-conflict situations. This needs to be given the formal recognition it deserves.

One of the major problems facing organizations charged with disaster management is gross lack of funds. The Honourable Minister for Works and Housing in 2002 admitted that the Federal Fire Service needs as much ₦4.6 billion to put it in proper shape i.e. effective and functional. Activities of most NGOs involved in disaster management especially as regards rescue and responses are also hampered by inadequate funds. The Nigeria Red Cross Society seems to fare better because of financial and logistic support it receives from the IRCS. Even when funds are made available, improper coordination between stakeholders in disaster management, especially in response and rescue, is inefficient and ineffective. There was the case in May 2002 when the warehouse of NEMA in Lagos went up in flames. Improper coordination resulted in insufficient water supply that rendered the ill equipped (vehicle, equipment and manpower) fire service impotent, thereby allowing relief materials worth millions of Naira to be gutted by fire. The effective coordination and networking mandate of NEMA can only be achieved when it is properly funded, monitored and evaluated, albeit periodically.

The commitment and sincerity of various tiers of government, especially the federal government poses a bottleneck to effective conflict/emergency management. Due to incessant change in the administration of the country in the past years, government policies and guidelines were never continuous or stable. While some governments see conflict/disaster management purely from a relief point of view others perceive it purely from the rehabilitation viewpoint. This narrow focus inhibits development and affects broader issues like post-conflict health delivery, the focus of this study, adversely. There is also the logistic problem in disaster/conflict management in Nigeria. The requisite equipment that is necessary for effective responses and rescue is not in place. For instance, effective communication gadgets warning/alert signals, disaster forecasting tools, like early-warning models, etc are lacking. However, the situation has improved slightly with the recent GSM revolution in Nigeria.

Inadequate capacity building and training in anticipation of conflict/disaster situations is totally absent in the country. A case in point is the January 2002 bomb blast in Lagos, which resulted in the drowning of many of the victims in canals. It was impossible to get professional divers to assist in the rescue operation because the country apparently has little or none of them at all. Rather local fishermen were credited for the rescue operation. However, if the NDRP is effectively implemented in respect of capacity building, it should be possible to improve on the lack of adequate human capital. But Nigeria seems to have a good start through the two training programmes at the Master's level in the Institute of African Studies and CEPACS, both in University of Ibadan; and at the diploma level in LASU. There are also opportunities for collaboration in peace and conflict research in the country. For example, AREF has promoted one such centre in LASU while CEPACS collaborates with the Initiative on Conflict Resolution and Ethnicity (INCORE), University of Ulster, Derry/Londonderry, Northern Ireland in research and organization of conferences, seminars and workshops. In spite of this seeming progress, there is still lack of training capacity for NGO officials mostly involved in post-conflict health care in the country and the West African subregion.

More importantly, in spite of the existence of a Department of Relief and Rehabilitation in NEMA, its activities, as enunciated in the NDRP, are focused mainly at the short-term relief end. Besides, we found out that neither NEMA nor NCFR and in fact the FMOH has any unit that coordinates the activities of NGOs, particularly NNGOs, to ensure that there is no duplication, wastages and redundancies in health care delivery in under-conflict and in post-conflict situations. Also, our study did not reveal the existence of any guidelines or other instruments to do this. This will mean that the critical dilemmas of post conflict health care identified by Macrae (1997) may be difficult to contain in Nigeria.

14.1.8 *The Role of ECOWAS in Post-Conflict Health Care*

At inception, ECOWAS aimed at harmonizing and coordinating national policies as well as promoting integration programmes, projects and activities of all its member states in about twenty sectors including health. In particular, a subsection of one of its articles (Article 61) enjoined member states to encourage and strengthen cooperation in health matters. Besides, Articles 58(2) of the Revised Treaty addressed explicit issues of conflict resolution. However, while protocols on Non-Agression by member states and on Mutual Assistance on Defence between member states have been in existence for a long time, it was only in December 1999 that Heads of State and Government of the community ratified the protocol on the mechanism for conflict Prevention, Management, Resolution and Peace-keeping and Security, in 'Lome, Togo.

The West African Health Organization (WAHO) whose treaty was signed in Abuja, Nigeria on 9th July, 1987 is empowered by Article 2 of its protocol to takeoff through the merger of two subregional health organizations, which were originally serving Anglophone and Francophone West Africa, respectively. The West African Health Community(WAHC) is the subregional health organization serving Anglophone West Africa while *Organisation de coordination et de Cooperation pour la Lutte contre les Grandes Endemies*(OCCGE) serves Francophone countries except the Republic of Guinea. WAHO is expected to serve all ECOWAS Member States, i.e. all five Anglophone countries, all ten Francophone countries and the two Lusaphone countries of Guinea-Bissau and Cape Verde. The objective of WAHO 'shall be the attainment of the highest possible standard and protection of the health of the peoples in the subregion, harmonization of the policies of Member States, pooling of resources, cooperation with one another and with others for a collective and strategic combat against the health problems of the subregion'. However, of the fourteen functions assigned to WAHO, only one is explicitly linked to health care delivery under conflict. Even then, there does not seem to be any explicit concern for solving health problems arising from violent conflict except in as much as they only cause 'emergencies'.

The establishment of a Mechanism for Conflict Prevention, Management, Resolution, Peace-keeping and Security (MCPMRPS), by ECOWAS marked another milestone in the life of the Community. This was formalized in a more enduring fashion with the establishment of ECOMOG (ECOWAS Cease-fire Monitoring Group), and the subregional intervention in the late 1980s to stem the tide of the ensuing civil war in Liberia. In addition to this development, sixteen Heads of State and Government of ECOWAS signed the, *Declaration of Moratorium on the Importation, Exportation and Manufacture of Light Weapons in West Africa* on 31st October, 1998. This moratorium, commonly known as the West African Small Arms Moratorium(WASAM), became effective on 1st November, 1998 for a renewable period of three years. It is an innovative approach for peace-building and conflict-prevention. Though, not a legally-binding regime, it is an expression of shared political will.

While ECOWAS can be said to have a good beginning in conflict management so far, however a lot of emphasis is laid on the military aspect. The community has also given some consideration to the management of relief and human activities, under which health care delivery under conflict as well as post conflict situations implicitly fall. But the regulations of ECOMOG do not give explicit consideration to health care delivery in conflict and post-conflict situations, beyond that of its officials. This is a big limitation in ECOWAS legislation which needs a revisit.

However, the protocol establishing MCPMRPS recognizes ECOMOG as one of its three main institutions. The good news is that this protocol has also broadened the structure of ECOMOG to include civilian and military modules of member states, which can be called for deployment as and when needed. Its roles and functions can therefore be creatively broadened to include health care delivery under conflict and post-conflict situations. In this connection, such roles as: humanitarian intervention in support of humanitarian disaster; preventive deployment; and any other operations; should be mandated by the Mediation and Security Council of MCPMRPS.

Using WACH as a case study to evaluate the state of readiness of the health institutions of ECOWAS for post-conflict health care delivery, our study found that at present, the agency appears inadequate to address issues relating to health care delivery under conflict and/or in post-conflict situations. However, it has features and characteristics like training, research and information dissemination infrastructure as well as specialized human capacity, that can be adopted and adapted for building the necessary institutional framework for health care delivery in under-conflict and in post-conflict situations. Thus, ECOWAS and its agencies as presently constituted are not well equipped to deal with the problems and challenges posed by health care delivery under conflict. In recent times, particularly with the adoption of the MCPMRPS Protocol, there is a window of opportunity for adapting the existing framework to face these challenges.

14.2 Implications of the Study and Recommendations

West African countries are poor and conflict has made them poorer. One major implication of this study is that conflict prevention, management and resolution is very important in the promotion of development and reduction of poverty in the subregion. In this connection, the study recommends that the regional approach to doing this, which has already begun at the level of ECOWAS, should be implemented and strengthened. This will be highlighted more fully later on in this section.

At the national level, all the study countries were found to spend minimally on health compared to other favoured sectors like defence. It is recommended that government should endeavour to improve the financing of health care both in peacetime and during conflict. Efforts already developed to improve the funding of health care delivery by all stakeholders using the instrumentality of health reforms, needs to be sustained.

In conflict countries, the negative effects on the health system, particularly health infrastructure and supply of health personnel complicated the problems of shortages in the system, including finance. All the countries that were studied relied heavily on outside assistance particularly through NGOs, yet many did not have relevant agencies, policies and guidelines for health care delivery under conflict. The implication is that all the countries do not have a proactive approach to healthcare delivery under conflict and in post-conflict situations. In particular, there is no way of coordinating the activities of NGOs to ensure that there is no duplication of efforts, wastages and redundancies. In the non-conflict countries of Cote d'Ivoire and Nigeria, the condition is somehow different. There is some framework on the ground for health care delivery under emergency/conflict but they need to be adapted for more effective post-conflict health care delivery. However, in none of these countries is there any effective system on the ground for coordinating the activities of NGOs to avoid duplication, wastages and redundancies. The result is that in the entire subregion, any interventions on health care delivery under conflict and in post-conflict situations will not be sustainable and the critical dilemmas of post-conflict health care enunciated by Macrae (1997) cannot be contained.

This study therefore recommends that countries of West Africa should make deliberate efforts to develop the necessary institutional and legal framework for health care under conflict and in post-conflict situations. This should include the framework for coordinating the activities of NGOs to ensure the sustainability of their interventions. Efforts at conflict resolution, prevention and management at the regional level, should be directed at improving post-conflict health care delivery. For example, it is gratifying that the protocol establishing MCPMRPS explicitly recognizes the contributions of civilians to peace keeping. This makes it easy to explicitly consider the problems of post-conflict health care delivery under this initiative. It will be

178

necessary, however to revise the ECOMOG regulations to take into cognizance this broadened outlook of ECOMOG as an agent of Conflict Prevention, Management, Resolution, Peace-keeping and Security.

Overall, we propose that ECOWAS should adopt a holistic and coordinated approach to health care delivery in under-conflict and post-conflict situations in which post-conflict rehabilitation is done within the general framework of political-social-economic rehabilitation. This will ensure that the three dilemmas of legitimacy, sustainability and coherence are taken care of almost simultaneously. Political rehabilitation will ensure the legitimacy of the transitional government. A holistic approach will also ensure that all the dimensions of relief-rehabilitation-development continuum will be taken into consideration with a view to ensuring that the necessary caveat of bringing about sustainability is taken care of. Of course, cohesion will be assured because, right from the outset, the programme will be coordinated, ensuring that there is no duplication of efforts and the actions and action plans focus on the needs of the affected populations and systems, and that what is provided is not just what the donors want to give, but what the country desires.

The good news is that the MCPMRPS adopts this holistic approach which recognizes the importance of the political, social and economic dimensions of post-conflict management. The Authority, the Security Council; and the Executive Secretariat, as well as their three organs: the Defence and Security Commission; the Council of Elders and ECOMOG provide adequate institutional framework, which can be creatively adapted, together with a proactive WAHO, if and when it decides to address the challenges posed by healthcare delivery under conflict and post-conflict situations in West Africa health care delivery.

However, ECOWAS will need to wake up from its stupor and implement the protocol of WAHO, but with an explicit mandate on the management of health care under conflict and post-conflict situations. WAHO and its component agencies will need to be strengthened organizationally and financially to be able to carry out this additional but important responsibility. It will need to go beyond 'routine' training of specialist health personnel to giving specialized training in health care provision under conflict and post-conflict situations. The colleges of WAHC and OCCGE can easily be adapted to do this critical assignment, perhaps with technical assistance from identified donor agencies and institutions, particularly using short-term training techniques.

In this connection, the problem of non-availability of training programmes for capacity development in health care delivery under conflict will need to be given wider consideration beyond what WAHO can do. Our study showed that until recently, there is no university in the subregion that has any programme in peace and conflict studies, in general. Besides, we are not aware of any training programme so far in health care delivery under conflict and in post-conflict situations in particular.

179

The training programmes identified in Nigeria: two Master's programmes in the Institute of African Studies and CEPACS all in the University of Ibadan; and the diploma programme in LASU, Lagos will need adaptation to take into consideration the needs of post-conflict health care in Nigeria and in the West African subregion. The CEPACS programme has already students from all over Africa including Sierra Leone, Liberia, Sudan, and Cameroon, among others. In addition, in conjunction with WAHO, these institutions can develop short-term training courses to meet the requirements of the subregion in health care delivery under conflict.

14.3   Limitations of the Study

One of the major limitations of the study stems from the way its data were collected. It was planned to use a random sample of the health facilities studied, stratified by ownership and location. This was fairly possible in Sierra Leone and to some extent Liberia (though there was over-sampling of government facilities). In Guinea-Bissau, this was not possible. This can affect the comparability of the results. Accordingly, the study adopted a case study approach in its analysis. This will at least afford us the opportunity to gain insight into the extent to which conflict has affected the health systems of the study countries. Besides, it should be able to dramatize the enormity of the problems faced by conflict countries with a view to bringing these to the attention of those who can assist. In spite of this limitation, it is our considered view that the results of the study have dramatized the direction as well as given some estimates of the extent of the impact of conflict on health care delivery in West Africa.

There is a general lack of financial data at the facility level in many of the health facilities surveyed. In many cases, the averages used were computed from a small proportion of the respondents. This makes the generalizability of the results difficult. In spite of this, the analysis done was also able to give an insight into the direction of shortage of funds, if not the magnitude, and demonstrated how this affected health care delivery.

The period of conflict varied from country to country. In two of the countries, conflict had ended completely when data were collected. In Sierra Leone, however, conflict was still on-going in a few of the facilities surveyed. The use of the recall method for data collection has its limitations for the reliability and accuracy of the estimates so derived, particularly in situations where record-keeping is very poor. The same situation applies in the case of this study.

14.4   Suggestions for Further Studies

This present study can be improved upon by conducting a study with improved methodology particularly in relation to data collection. Efforts should be made to ensure that better and more credible financial data are collected. Such studies can also employ more rigorous analytical, perhaps predictive techniques.

This study has also not evaluated the impact of post-conflict health care delivery on development. An area of future study relates to the impact of (in)active post-conflict health policy and delivery on the development process. The costs of conflict generally and that of health care under conflict, in particular, needs study. It has important policy implications, particularly in respect to policy choices. This is an area that deserves some research attention.

14.5   Concluding Remarks

This study examined the state of readiness of countries of West Africa for health care delivery under conflict and in post-conflict situations. It used three countries which experienced conflict in the late 1980s and/or the 1990s as well as two non-conflict countries, as case studies. For the regional dimension, it analyzed the potentials of ECOWAS and its institutions for health care delivery under conflict.

It was able to demonstrate that conflict had deleterious effects on the health system. Besides, it showed that countries of West Africa are generally not adequately prepared for health care delivery under conflict, both at national and regional levels, even though recent developments in ECOWAS, and Nigeria offer windows of opportunity of possible system adaptation to improve the response of the subregion to post-conflict health care. The study offered suggestions on how West Africa can proactively tackle the problems posed by conflict on its health systems.

---

[1] We note that for Liberia, as stated earlier, there were no socio-economic data in most international publications for the civil war years, and immediately thereafter; also a negative impact of the war. The period referred to in the case of Liberia was 1980, 1984 – 1987. For other countries, it was 1995 –2000.

[2] There were no comparative data for Liberia even in the earlier period chosen for study.

REFERENCES

African Development Bank. 1992. *Nigeria: Multi-State Health Rehabilitation Project – Appraisal Report.* Abidjan.

Ajayi, S. Ibi. 2002. *Institutions: The Missing Link in the Growth Process?* Presidential Address Delivered at the Annual Conference of the Nigerian Economic Society, 7 – 8 August. Nigerian Economic Society Secretariat, Ibadan,

Ball, Nicole. 1998. *Complex Crisis and Complex Peace: Humanitarian Coordination in Angola,* United Nations Office for the Coordination of Humanitarian Affairs, UNHCA On-line.

Barnes, Sam. 1998. NGOs in Peace-keeping Operations, their Role in Mozambique. *Development in Practice,* 8(3): 309-322.

Birch, Marion. 1999. Background and Rationale for the Continuation of the Health Transition Programme in Angola. Paper presented at the Workshop on Post-Conflict Health Policy and Planning, London School of Hygiene and Tropical Medicine, February 4-5.

Bond, G and J. Vincent. 1990. Living on the Edge: Changing Social Structures in the Context of AIDS. In Hansen and Twaddle(Eds.) *Changing Uganda: the Dilemmas of Structural Adjustment and Revolutionary Change.* James Currey, London; pp. 113 – 129.

Bush, Kenneth. 1998. *A Measure of Peace: Peace Impact Assessment (PCIA) of Development Projects in Conflict Zones.* Working Paper No 1, The Peace and Reconstruction Program Initiative, IDRC.

Development Assistance Committee (DAC). 1997. *DAC Guidelines on Conflict, Peace and Development Cooperation.* OECD, Paris.

Duffield, M. 1991. *War and Famine in Africa.* Oxfam Research Paper No 5. Oxfam Publications, Oxford.

ECOWAS .1992. ECOWAS Decisions on the Liberian Crisis. *Special Supplement from the Official Journal of ECOWAS* Vol. 21.

ECOWAS .1999. *Annual Report, 1998/99.* Abuja, Nigeria; October.

ECOWAS .2000a. *Annual Report.* Abuja, Nigeria; October.

ECOWAS. 2000b. *Economic Community of West African States, Silver Jubilee Anniversary: Achievements and Prospects 1975 – 2000.* ECOWAS, Abuja.

Eklund, P. and K. Staven. 1996. Community Health Insurance Through Prepayment Schemes in Guinea Bissau in Shaw, R. P. and Ainsworth (eds.). *Financing Health Services through User Fees and Insurance: Case Studies from Africa.* World Bank Discussion Papers, Africa Technical Department Series No. 294

Federal Ministry of Health. *1998. The National Health Policy to Achieve Health for all Nigerians.* Lagos.

Federal Ministry of Health. *2000. Health Sector Reform Medium Term Plan of Action 2001-2003.* Abuja.

Gertler, P. and Van der Gaag 1990. *The Willingness to Pay for Medical Care: Evidence from Two Developing Countries.* The Johns Hopkins University Press, London.

Hanlon, J. 1992. *Mozambique: Who Calls The Shorts?* James Currey, London.

Humblet, Pierre and M. Biot. 1999. MSF Programmes in Post-Conflict Situations. Paper presented at the Workshop on Post-Conflict Health Policy and Planning, London School of Hygiene and Tropical Medicine, February 4-5.

Kurmar, Krishmar. 1997. The Nature and Scope of International Assistance in Rebuilding War-Torn Societies. In Kumar, K.(ed.) *Rebuilding Societies after Civil War: Critical Roles for International Assistance.* Lynne Rienner, Boulder, Colorado

Lambo, Eyitayo. 2003. *Resource Mobilization for an Expanded and Comprehensive Response to HIV/AIDS and its Implications.* Commonwealth Regional Health Community Secretariat, Arusha, Tanzania.

Luxen, Jean-Pierre. 1997. *Relief-Rehabilitation-Development in the Field of Health: Proposed Guidelines for Action.* Health and Development Series Working Paper No 3, Directorate-General for Development, European Commission, Brussels.

Macrae, Joanne. 1997. Dilemmas of Legitimacy, Sustainability, and Coherence: Rehabilitating the Health Sector. In Kumar, K.(ed.) *Rebuilding Societies after Civil War: Critical Roles for International Assistance.* Lynne Rienner, Boulder, Colorado.

Macrae, Joanne, Anthony Zwi and Vivienne Forsythe. 1995a. Aid Policy in Transition: A Preliminary Analysis of 'Post'-Conflict Rehabilitation of the Health Sector, *Journal for International Development* 7(4): 669-684.

Macrae, Joanne, Anthony Zwi with Vivienne Forsythe. 1995b *Post-Conflict Rehabilitation: Preliminary Issues for Consideration by the Health Sector*. London School of Hygiene and Tropical Medicine, PHP Departmental Publication No. 16.

Mbanefoh, Gini F., Adedoyin Soyibo and John C. Anyanwu. Forthcoming. Health Care Financing in Nigeria: Federal State and Local Government Levels. In Germeno, Mwanbu, Joseph Wang' Ombe and Gasper Munishi (Eds). *Improving Health Policy in the Africa*, University of Nairobi, Nairobi.

MHSW. 2000. *National Health Policy: A Framework for Health Reform in the New Millennium*. Ministry of Health and Social Welfare, Monrovia.

NEMA. 2001. *National Disaster Response Plan.* National Emergency Mangement Agency, Abuja, Nigeria.

NEMA. 2000. Nigeria: Economic Policy and Strategy: The Way Forward. Abuja.

Ogbaji, Joseph O. 2003. Realigning National Laws and Obligations for Refugee Management: Nigerian Experiences. Paper Presented at the International Seminar marking the 2003 World Refugee Day, University of Ibadan, 20th June.

Olusola, Segun. 2003. The Role of National Commission for Refugees in the Management of Refugees and Internally Displaced Persons. Paper Presented at the International Seminar Commemorating the 2003 World Refugee Day, University of Ibadan, 20 June.

Pavignani, Enrico. 1999. The Reconstruction Process in the Health Sector in Mozambique. Paper presented at the Workshop on Post-Conflict Health Policy and Planning, London School of Hygiene and Tropical Medicine, February 4-5.

ROS. 1993. *National Health Policy*. Freetown, Republic of Sierra Leone Department of Health and Social Services, June.

ROS. 1994. *National Health Action Plan*. Freetown, Republic of Sierra Leone Department of Health and Social Services, February.

Seck, Jacqueline .1999. *West African Small Arms Moratorium: High-Level Consultations on the Modalities for the Implementation of PCASED*. United Nations Institute for Disarmament Research, Geneva and United Nations Regional Centre for Peace and Disarmament in Africa, Lome.

Siegel, B., Peters, D. and Kamara, S. 1996. *Health Reform in Africa: Lessons from Sierra Leone*. World Bank Discussion Paper No. 347

Smallman-Raymor, M. and A. Cliff. 1991. Civil War and the Spread of AIDS in Central Africa. *Epidemiology of Infectious Diseases* 107(1): 69 - 80.

Soyibo, Adedoyin.1998. *ECOWAS: So Long A Journey to EMU*. Working Paper 7, Development Policy Centre, Ibadan.

Soyibo, Adedoyin.1999. 'Post-Conflict' Health Policy and Planning in West Africa: What Roles for ECOWAS and Regional Health Institutions ? Paper presented at the Workshop on Post-Conflict Health Policy and Planning, London School of Hygiene and Tropical Medicine, February 4-5.

Soyibo, Adedoyin, *1998. Effectiveness of Social Expenditure on Poverty Alleviation in Nigeria*. Development Policy Centre, Ibadan, Working Paper 99/13.

Soyibo, Adedoyin, Gini F. Mbanefoh, John C. Anyawu. Forthcoming. Fiscal Decentralization in Nigeria: Have Health Expenditure Improved at the Local Level? in Germano Mwanbu and Joseph Wang'Ombe (Eds). *Health Policy Research in the Third World*, IHPP, Washington DC.

UN. 1998. *The Causes of Peace and Promotion of Durable Peace and Sustainable Development in Africa*. Report of the Secretary-General to the United Nations Security Council, 16 April.

UN. 2002. *World Population Prospects; The 2000 Revision, Volume III: Analytical Report*. United Nations, New York.

USAID, 1996. *Saving Lives Today and Tomorrow: A Decade Report on USAID Child Survival Program*. USAID, Washington, DC.

WHO. 1998. *Health Strategic Response: Relief, Rehabilitation and Development*. Report from a Meeting, 18-19 June, Geneva.

WHO. 2000. *World Health Report 2000*. World Health Organization, Geneva.

Wippman, D. 1993 Enforcing the Peace: ECOWAS and the Liberian Civil War, in L. F. Damrosch (ed.). *Enforcing Restraint: Collective Intervention in Internal Conflicts*, New York Council of Foreign Relations Press.

World Bank, 1994a. *Nigeria Social Sector Strategy Review*. World Bank, Washington DC.

World Bank, 1994b. *Better Health in Africa: Experience and Lesson Learned*. Washington DC.

World Bank, 1996. *Staff Appraisal Report: Republic of Sierra Leone, Integrated Health Sector Project*. World Bank Report No. 13947-SL.

Zwi, A. and A. Cabral. 1991. Identifying 'high risk situations' for Preventing AIDS. *British Medical Journal* 303: 1527-1529.

Zwi, A. and A. Ugalde. 1989. Towards an Epidemiology of Political Violence in the Third World. *Social Science and Medicine* 28(7): 633-642.

INDEX

Abuja Peace Accord, 10
Abuja Treaty, 29
Academic Community, 39
Act of Parliament, 171
African
- Development Bank (ADB), 98,168
- Refuge Foundation (AREF), 13, 134, 141, 172, 175
Aid Agencies, 6
AIDS, 24, 32, 45, 62, 133
Alibaloye, J.A.A., 135
Allo Docteurs, 170
Alma Ata Conference, 1978, 55
American Slaves, 28
Americo - Liberians (freed slaves), 28
Armed Conflicts, 3-4, 6
Armed Forces Revolutionary Council (AFRC), 148
Assembly of Health Ministers (AHM), 149
Association of African Universities, 13

Bedie, President, 40, 42
Bilateral
- Agencies, 56
- Organisations, 94
Biu, Brigadier, 111
Boigny, Houphet, 40

Care International, 168
Caritas Makeni, Care International, 97,139,168, 174
Catholica Nationale, 64, 165
Cease - fire agreements, 68
Centre for
- Disease Control (CDC), U.S., 57
- Peace and Conflict Studies (CEPACS), 13, 141, 175, 180
Cerebrospinal meningitis (CSM), 52
Child Nutrition, 44
Civic Conflicts, 15, 28
Civil War, 10, 21, 28-29, 34, 61-64, 66, 68-69, 80, 94, 127, 147, 166
- in Liberia, 177
Communal Violence in Nigeria, 139
Communicable Diseases,24, 31, 37, 62, 99, 168
Communication Gadgets, 141
Community-Based
- First aid (CBFA) projects, 121, 171
- Organisations (CBOs), 129, 171
Community Health Officers, 99-100, 168
Community-managed village Health Posts (USBs), 24-26, 63

Community Representative, 39
Conflict
- Emergency Management Agencies, 127
- Management and Rehabilitation, 8, 17-18
- Resolution, 176
    - Prevention and Management, 178
Connaught Hospital, 168
Control of Illicit Light Weapons Trafficking and Proliferation, 146
Council of
- Elders, 145, 152, 179
- Registered Engineers of Nigeria (COREN), 131
Country Health Teams (CHTs), 79-80, 94,167
Croix Rouge (Red Cross) of Côte d'Ivoire, 121, 170

Declaration of Moratorium on the Importation, Exportation and Manufacture of Light Weapons in West Africa, 177
Defence and Security Commission, 145, 152
Democratic Feudalism, 28
Department of
- Finance, 39
- Health, 38-39
Development Finance Institutions, 98, 168
Director of
- Help Operations, 116
- Medical Services, 116
Disaster
- Forecasting Tools, 141
- Management Services, 174-175
    - Bodies, 129
Doctors for all Nations, 134, 172
Donor Agencies, 7, 87, 98-99, 139, 165, 174
Donor Community, 39
Drug-resistant Malaria, 160

Ecological Fund, 128
Economic Community of West African States (ECOWAS), 5-7, 33, 48, 68, 142-153, 176-179, 181
- Cease-Fire Monitoring Group (ECOMOG), 10, 18, 33, 144, 146-149, 152-153, 177, 179
Emergency Health Services, 119
Environmental Degradation, 128
Ethnic
- Antagonism, 48
- Composition of Liberia, 28
- Conflicts, 48
- Groups, 13, 40, 48
- Rivalries, 40
- Tension, 115

187

Ethno-religious and other communal crises, 127
European
- Colonialism, 28
- Development Fund, 116, 170
- Union, 41, 116, 170
External Dept Payment, 50

Family
- Planning Services, 53
- Reunion, 133
Federating Units, 48
Federal
- and State Fire Services, 138
- Environmental Protection Agency
Decree, 1989, 128
- Medical Centres, 133
- Ministry of Health (FMOH), 54-55, 57,
131, 134, 138, 141, 172, 174, 176
- Road Safety Act, 128
- Road Safety Corps, 128, 138, 174
Female Genital Mutilation, 121, 171
Fire Brigade, 169-170
First Aid Health Care Services, 116, 169

Gbagbo, Laurent, 41
Geneva Convention, 1951, 139
Global Warming, 128
Government
- Agencies, 121-125, 128, 171
- of Liberia (GOL) 81-82, 94-95, 167
- of the Republic of Sierra Leone
(GOROS), 98-99, 168
Gross
- Domestic
- Investment (GDI), 21, 30, 50
- Product (GDP), 21, 29-30, 33-35, 38,
41-42, 44, 49-50, 157-159
- Savings (GNS), 29
- National
- Income, 21, 40, 50
- Investment, 157-158
- Savings (GNS), 21, 29, 34, 50, 157-158
- Public Investment (GPI), 21, 34, 50
Groupement des Sapeurs Pompiers Militaries
(GSPM) - Fire brigade, 115-121, 125,
169-170
GSM Revolution in Nigeria, 141, 175
Guei, Robert, 40-41

Health and Population Project, 98
Health
- Care financing, 98
- Centres (clinics), 24
- Distribution, 76,93, 110
- Expenditure, 76

- Finance reforms, 98
- Financing, 12, 15-16
- Information Management System, 14, 111
- Level (Disability-Adjusted Life
Expectancy)(DALE), 76, 93, 110
- Plan 1976, 68, 77, 166
- Professionals, 39, 81, 86-87, 102-103, 144
- Reforms, 39, 178
- Resources, 163
- Sector Reform (HSR), 55
- Services Coordinating Committee (HSCC),
79-80, 93-94, 167
- Status, 158-159
- System, 3, 6-7, 10, 13-14, 17, 29, 34,
46, 49, 53, 61-62, 68-69, 72, 76,
81-84, 99-100, 110, 160-161,
166-168, 178, 181
- System Development Project (HSDP)
Implementation Plan, 55, 57
- System Fund (HSF), 56
- System Programmes, 56
Highway Ambulance Services, 133
HIV/AIDS, 24, 31-32, 37, 45, 52-53, 55-57,
62, 121, 144, 171
- Program Development Aide Memo ire,
56-57
HIV Infection, 12
Human Capital, 164
Human Resource Base, 12-13
- Capacity Development, 17
- Development, 6
Human
- Resources, 14, 85-87, 102-103, 120
- Resources Development Plan (HRDP), 38
Humanitarian
- and Refugee Studies, 13
- Emergencies, 115

ICRC, 123-124
IMF, 41
Immunization, 133
Infant Mortality Rate, 31, 35
Infectious diseases, 31, 36, 44, 51, 77, 159-160
Initiative on Conflict Resolution and Ethnicity
(INCORE), 141, 175
Institute of African Studies, 13, 141, 175, 180
Institutional Reforms, 16
Internally Displaced Persons (IDPs), 139, 174
International
- Affairs, 3
- Agencies, 6, 166
- Community, 3, 41, 112
International Development Administration
(IDA), 57

International
- Donor agencies, 174
- Federation, 123
  - and National Society, 121-122
    of Red Cross and Red Crescent Societies
    (IFRC), 122, 124, 170
- Law, 18
- Organisations, 63, 77
- Publications, 93
- Red Cross and Red Crescent
  Societies (IFRC), 129, 132, 139,
  171-172, 174
Intra-state Armed Conflicts, 3
Ivorian Political Scenery, 41

Kabbah, Tejan President, 33, 148
Koromah, Johnny Paul, 148

Lagos State University (LASU), 13, 173, 175,
  180
Least Developed Countries, 84
Leaones and Cents, 97, 168
Level of Security, 9
Liberian
- Civil war, 28, 80, 90
- Economy, 29, 157
- Refugee operation, 123
- Refugees, 139
Life expectancy, 23, 30, 43, 50, 158-159
Lions' Club, 117
Local Government Health Offices, 133
Local
- Resource mobilization, 166
- Wars, 3
l' ordre de Malte, 170

Maternal and Child Health (MCH) Services, 53
Maternal Mortality Rate, 30, 44, 50, 62, 158-159
Maternity and Infant Protection Centre(MIP),
  46-47
Mechanism for Conflict Prevention, Management
  Resolution, Peacekeeping and Security
  (MCPMRPS), 144-145, 148-149, 152,
  176-177, 179
Mediation and Security Council, 145, 152
Medical Research Ethics, 97
Military
- Action, 12
- Health services, 45
- Regime, 28, 42, 102
Ministry of
- Defence, 119
- Health, 14, 16, 25, 47, 117, 166
  - and Sanitation, 97, 110, 112, 168
  - and Social Welfare (MHSW), 79-83,
    93-94, 167

- Public Health Survey, 46
- National Education and Scientific
  Research, 47
- Public Health (MINSAP), 26-27, 61, 63,
  77, 166-167
Mother clubs, 133
Multilateral
- Agencies, 4, 56
- Organisations, 17, 94
Mutual Assistance on Defence, 176

National
- Action Committee on AIDS (NACA), 56
- Blood Transfusion Centre, 45
- Boundaries, 4
- Commission for Refugees (NCFR),
  138-139, 174, 176
- Committee on Ecological Problems, 127
- Committee on Emergency Preparedness
  and Response, 133, 172
- Council for Rehabilitation, 135
- Council of Health, 54
- Disaster Response Plan (NDRP), 134,
  136-138, 141, 173-175
- Emergency Management Agency (NEMA)
  128-132, 134, 136-138,
  140-141, 171-176
- Emergency Relief Agency (NERA), 128,
  135, 140, 171
- Health Action Plan (NHAP), 37, 99-100,
  110-111, 168-169
- Health Development Plan (NHDP), 46-47
- Health Management Information
  System (NHMIS), 57
- Health Policy (NIIP), 36, 47, 53, 55, 79,
  81-82, 99-100, 110-111, 167-169
- Health System, 79
- Health Workers' Training Institute, 45
- Identity Card, 41
- Office of Civil Protection (ONPC), 116
- Patriotic Front of Liberia (NPFL), 29
- Population Policy, 46
- Provisional Ruling Council (NPRC), 33
- Public Health Laboratory, 45
- Public Hygiene Institute, 45
- Refugee Camps, 139
- Social Contingency Funds, 45
- Societies, 121-122, 171
- Vision 2010 Report, 55
New Law Provisions for the Health System, 79
Nigeria
- Armed Forces, 128, 171
- Fire Service, 128, 171
- Police Force, 128, 137, 171
- Red Cross and Red Crescent Society, 133

- Security and Civil Defence Corps, 138, 174

Nigerian
- Air Force Disaster Response Units, 138, 171
- Army, 138, 174
- Civil War (1967- 1970), 128, 171
- Red Cross Society (NRCS), 127, 129, 131-132, 137, 171-174
- Society of Engineers (NSE), 131
Non
- Communicable Diseases, 24, 52
- Governmental Organisations (NGOs) 4-5, 7, 13-17, 53, 56, 61, 68 74-81, 84, 94-96, 99, 101, 104, 110, 112, 121-126, 128-129, 131-134, 139-141, 164-172, 174-176, 178
- Role of, 74-76, 90-93, 107-109
- Health professionals, 102 -103
Northern NGOs (NNGOs), 17, 93, 95, 166, 176
Nwokodie, S.C., 135

OAU Convention, 1969, 139
Obasanjo, President, 55
Olowu, Oluremi, 135
Olusola, Segun, 134, 172
Onobare, Timothy, 135
Organisation de coordination et de
- Cooperation pour la Lutte contre les Grandes Endemies (OCCGE), 143-144, 152, 176, 179
Organized Private Sector, 129
ORSEC Plan (Plan ORSEC), 115-116, 169
Ouattara, Alassane Dramane, 40-41
Overseas Development Assistance (ODA), 167

Pan-American Health Organisation (PAHO), 144
Paris Agreement, 10
Peace
- Agreement, 9
- and conflict studies, 13
- and security studies, 5
Peripheral Health Units (PHUs), 38
Physical Infrastructure, 12, 15
Planned Parenthood Association of Sierra Leone 97, 168
Point of Contact Management, 130
Policy and Management, 12-14
Political
- Asylum, 94
- Authourities, 41
- Committees. 26
- Factors, 11
- History, 33

- Instability, 115
- Landscape, 127
- Leaders, 40
- Rehabilitation, 151, 179
- Rivals, 40
- Tension, 28, 40
- Turmoil, 42
- Uncertainty, 14
- Will, 144, 146, 168
Population transition, 93
Post-conflict Health
- Care 62-63, 77
- Delivery 4-7, 9, 79, 94, 96, 112, 157, 167, 181
- Policy, 12
- Impacts of 12-16
- Reforms 38-39
- Rehabilitation, 126
- System, 162
Post Disaster Management, 130
Post-emergency Rehabilitation Activities, 123
Post-war Health Budgets, 81, 94, 167
Pre-disaster Management, 130
Pre-war Budgets, 81, 94, 167
Preventive Health Care Services, 45
Primary Health Care (PHC), 17, 38, 55-56, 62 100, 167
- Programmes, 53-54
Prison Health Programme, 133
Professional Institutions, 167
Programme for the Coordination and Assistance for Security and Development (PCASED), 146
Protocol, 1967, 139
Public Health, 14, 168
Public Health
- and Population Ministry, 47
- Expenditure, 35
- Ministry, 45-46
- Pharmacy, 45

Rassemblement des Republicains (RDR) Party, 124
Reconciliation Forum, 41
Red
- Crescent Society, 170
- Cross and Red Crescent Society, 122, 124, 172
- Cross of Côte d'Ivoire (RCCI), 123-125
- Plan (Plan rouge), 115-116, 169
Refugee camps. 174
Regional
- Health institutions, 6-7
- Instability. 4
- Peace and security issues, 147

190

Relief
- and/or rehabilitation programme, 10
- Reconstruction and rehabilitation
continuum, 76
- Rehabilitation and reconstruction, 4-7
- Rehabilitation development continuum
139, 144, 151, 179
Responsiveness
- Distribution, 76, 110
- Level, 76, 110
Revolutionary United Front (RUF), 148, 164
Rouge, Khmer, 10
Rwandan genocide, 134, 172

Sankoh, Fode, 148
Save the Children of Sierra Leone, 97, 168
Secondary Health Care (SCH), 53-55
Self-employment Schemes, 139
Service d'Aide Medicale d'Urgence (SAMU) i.e.
Emergency Medical Help Service
115-121, 169-170
Sexual and Reproductive Health, 55
Sexually Transmitted Diseases (STDs), 12, 62
Sierra Leone Red Cross Society, 97, 168
Siera Leonean Civil War, 93
Sos Medecins, 170
- and Allo Docteurs and l ordre de Malte,
121
Specialist and Teaching Hospitals, 53
Staff Training, 77
State
- Emergency Management Committee,
130, 172
- Hospitals Management Board (SHMB), 54
- Ministry of Health (SMOH), 54
- Police Force, 116
Strasser, Valentine E.M., 102, 111
Street Riots, 41
Support Services Areas (SSAs), 137-138
System Responsiveness
- Distribution, 93
- Level, 93

Taylor, Charles, 10, 29, 73, 93-94
Technical Advisory Committee (TAC), 79, 94,
167
Terms of Trade, 157
Tertiary Health Care, 53-54, 84
Trade Balance, 22, 50
Traditional Birth Attendants (TBAs), 26

Uk Department for International
Development(DFID), 57
UN agencies, 123
UNDP, 63, 77, 146, 166
UNHCR, 124

UNITA, 10
United Nations
- Children's fund (UNICEF)
57, 63-64, 72, 77 79, 94, 98,
133, 139, 165--168, 172, 174
- Observer Mission in Sierra Leone
(UNOMSIL), 148
- Regional Centre for peace and
Disarmament in Africa, 146
United States
- Agency for International Development
(USAID), 57
- Departments of Labour and Defense, 57
University of Ibadan (U.I), 13, 180

Vieira, Joao Bernardo, 68, 148
Village Health
- Posts (USBs), 63, 66, 77, 166
- Workers (VHW), 25-27, 63, 166
Village Midwives, 25, 63, 77
Voluntary Organisations, 129
Vulnerability and Capacity Assessment, 122

War-related Health
- Conditions, 163
- Indications, 106
- Problems, 101
Warning Alert Signals, 141
Waste Disposal Decree, 1988, 128
West African
- College of
- Nursing, 150
- Physicians, 150
- Surgeons, 150
- Health
- Community (WAHC), 143,149-150,
152, 176-177, 179
- Organisation (WAHO), 5, 143-144,
152-153, 176, 179-180
-National Red Cross
- and Red Crescent Society, 121
- Societies, 121, 170
- Pharmaceutical Federation, 150
- Small Arms Moratorium (WASAM),
145-146, 177
World
- Bank, 35, 37-38, 41, 44, 48, 51, 56, 98, 168
- Food programme, 125
- Health Organisation (WHO), 57, 63-64
72, 77, 79, 93-94, 116, 133,
165-168, 170
- Health Accounts (NHA), 98
- World Health Report, 76

Zone d'Accrueil des Refugies (ZAR), 125